Dosage

Dosage

A Guiding Principle
for Health Communicators

J. David Johnson

ROWMAN & LITTLEFIELD PUBLISHERS, INC.
Lanham • Boulder • New York • Toronto • Plymouth, UK

Published by Rowman & Littlefield Publishers, Inc.
A wholly owned subsidiary of The Rowman & Littlefield Publishing Group, Inc.
4501 Forbes Boulevard, Suite 200, Lanham, Maryland 20706
www.rowman.com

10 Thornbury Road, Plymouth PL6 7PP, United Kingdom

British Library Cataloguing in Publication Information Available

Library of Congress Cataloging-in-Publication Data

Johnson, J. David.
  Dosage : a guiding principle for health communicators / J. David Johnson.
    p. ; cm.
  Includes bibliographical references.
  ISBN 978-1-4422-2124-6 (cloth : alk. paper) — ISBN 978-1-4422-2125-3 (pbk. : alk.
paper) — ISBN 978-1-4422-2126-0 (electronic)
  I. Title.
  [DNLM: 1. Interdisciplinary Communication. 2. Professional-Patient Relations. 3.
Information Dissemination. W 62]
  R727.3
  610.69'6—dc23   2013016918

Printed in the United States of America

To old ghosts, Steve Kinghorn and John Klett,
taken in a war beyond fathoming
that was enough for me.

Contents

Figures and Tables

TABLES

FIGURES

• 1 •

Introduction and Overview

PROLOGUE

$\mathcal{L}$et us examine the situation where a doctor is determining the dosage needed to treat a patient with thyroid cancer. Unconsciously in most situations, consciously if the physician is a particularly good one, at the same time that medical dosages are being determined, the physician is addressing underlying communication dosage problems in deciding how best to impart critical information to the patient (see table 1.1).

We are all somewhat familiar with the elements that would be considered when a doctor considers the dosage of a therapeutic agent. The physician will need to determine staging before more precise treatment protocols can be developed. If this is one of the diseases where personalized medicine is possible, the physician will need to do additional testing to determine the characteristics of the patient and whether they are predisposed to the delivery of various agents. The physician will have to consider the amount of the medicine to be given after surgical removal; how frequently the medicine will be given and for what duration, whether it's best to deliver the medicine intravenously or by pill; if radiation should be followed by chemotherapy and then by hormone therapy; if the medicine might potentially interact with other therapeutic agents the patient is being given; and whether or not there are factors relating to the patient, such as age, gender, underlying medical conditions, and so forth, that contraindicate the chemotherapy s/he has selected. The physician also needs to be concerned about the dysfunctional consequences of any therapies s/he has selected, including such issues as nausea, hair loss, disfigurement, tracheostomy; and so on.

1

Table 1.1. Dosage in a Medical Encounter

	Context	
Dosage Elements	*Medical*	*Communication*
Amount	Milligrams	Duration of face-to-face meeting
Frequency	Weekly for two months	Follow-ups
Sequencing	Radiation, then chemotherapy, then hormone therapy	Give diagnosis, next meeting details
Delivery systems	Intravenous Pill	Brochure, videotape, face-to-face
Interactions	Other medicines	Friends, family, support groups, Internet
Contraindications	Personalized medicine	Dementia
Dysfunctions	Side effects	Life circumstances

Coincident with his/her medical decision making, a set of decisions are reached relating to how all of this will be communicated to the patient with the resulting meaning the "therapeutic agent" that produces the desired effect. Unfortunately for both the physician and the patient, there is not the wealth of research evidence to guide this set of decisions that there is to guide medical decision making. The physician may decide to set aside a double appointment to discuss thoroughly all of the treatment options with the patient based on past experience and findings in health communication literature. Alternatively, s/he might decide to give the patient the diagnosis based on the medical tests; then, after the patient has had time to digest this bad news, to arrange for further testing to see if the cancer has spread, which will determine staging and associated treatments; then to follow up with a more lengthy, detailed interview in which treatment options after surgery are discussed. While this would be his/her preferred approach with most patients, the physician might also consider for older patients who suffer from dementia (a contraindication) that it would be best to have this sort of discussion with caregivers rather than the patients themselves. For most patients, the physician then decides what communication channels would be the most appropriate to supplement his/her face-to-face interview to deliver the message to the patient. S/he might decide to refer the patient to a website, to give the patient a brochure, to show the patient a videotape, and so forth. Unfortunately, the physician may not know how the information s/he has provided might interact with other information sources the patient is exposed to, such as friends and family, religious institutions, support groups, providers of alternative therapies and herbal remedies, and so on. The physician also needs to be concerned with how this might impact patients more broadly. In this case s/he might be worried about patients' history of depression and suicidal thoughts; their recent loss of a spouse; their continued unemployment;

and on and on. In short, for the medical treatment to be most effective, the physician needs to follow a parallel sequence relating to communication dosages to the one they follow more overtly for medical ones.

OVERVIEW

As the preceding example details, when confronted with problems in our everyday lives, we must decide how much effort we will engage in to achieve our ends. So, lovers must decide the best timing for telling their partners it is over. Marketing directors must decide how much TV time they should buy, how frequently to sell a product. Salesmen must decide when they have made enough arguments to close the deal, adapting their persuasive attempts to the level of resistance they sense in their audience. Surgeons must decide how much information they need to impart to their surgical team to deal with emergencies. Surgical technicians need to ensure that they get the right instrument for the next stage of the operation. Doctors, as in the preceding example, must realize that their means of delivery can stir up needless "allergies" to their proposed treatment by stimulating emotional reactions to their message. Teachers must decide whether a simple lecture will do or they will need exercises, as well as class discussion, to get a point across. Fundamentally, in our day-to-day interactions with others, we must constantly confront issues of dosage.

Here we will look at dosage metaphorically. When I am sick, I go to a doctor for a diagnosis. The doctor evaluates my condition and then prescribes a treatment. If I am a bad patient, I do not follow his/her prescription as to agency, frequency, duration, and so on, exactly. So I inadvertently skip doses, change treatment agents (often because of expense, the advice of friends, or just reverting to habits), and do not continue administration after the symptoms are gone.

In spite of decades of research on communication, we have at best only a fuzzy notion of what "dosage" is needed for particular effects. What amount of communication do we need to achieve particular purposes? Communication theories typically paint a picture of the pervasiveness of communication. Systems theories dwell on the importance of coordination and interdependence; interpretive theories focus on sharing of perspectives in sense-making activities, discourse theories on the importance of dialog for collective action, participation theories on the involvement of workers and so on.

These approaches embed the "communication metamyth" that more is better, with people always desiring more communication regardless of how much they are receiving (Zimmerman, Sypher, & Haas, 1996); interpersonal scholars historically argued that increased communication leads to "relational panacea" (Stafford, 2005, pp.107); and uncertainty reduction has often been cast as a "direct and linear function of an objective quantity of information" (Afifi & Afifi, 2009, p. 1).

Here I will argue that the metaphor of dosage offers a rich organizing principle for health communicators. It focuses our efforts on such fundamental, pragmatic communication issues as amount, frequency, sequencing, delivery system, interaction with other agents, and contraindications. It suggests compelling answers to fundamental problems that all health communicators must face. It is in the ultimate hope for the more complete development of the dosage metaphor that we look at some old problems, which are critical to any practitioner, with a new set of tools and vocabulary.

DOSAGE AND METAPHOR

As in medical treatments, the key question is just what "dosage" is needed. What proportion of people and what amount of communication are needed to achieve threshold and/or critical mass effects for social media? It may be the case that for a number of applications, minimalist communication strategies, involving some mediated communication and intense interpersonal communication involving only those immediately affected, may be the best approach or, alternatively, perhaps a more viral marketing approach targeting opinion leaders. Surprisingly there is little interest, or perhaps even awareness, that we really have only very limited knowledge of such a basic issue, one that every practicing health communicator must confront in one way or another.

We do not have measured approaches to problems. We do not know when to stop, and perhaps like a doctor who gives someone a drug because they expect one, in our consultant roles we are often pressed to do something. The dosage metaphor offers an encompassing way of addressing these issues, particularly with an emphasis on the increasing importance of outcomes in this age of accountability. It focuses on the issue of how much should I give, how often, for how long, with an underlying appreciation for the darker side of effects (e.g., overdoses, allergic reactions, contraindications) as well. The dosage metaphor has rich theoretic implications that also bridge us to persistent problems that practitioners face daily.

Metaphors become a way of seeing and thinking about life; they provide a way of understanding one thing by appeal to another. They have been central to our thinking about health organizations, such as hospitals, given their complexity. This was particularly so early on for issues related to productivity, efficiency, and effectiveness, seemingly the most rational of pursuits. Some of this early work on efficiency likened organizations to machines, while later work, more concerned with fit, match, and effectiveness, used more organismic metaphors.

Fundamentally dosage refers to the administration of a therapeutic agent in prescribed amounts. Given its ubiquity in medical disciplines, it is somewhat surprising that dosage has not been related in a more systematic way to health communication. Common definitions of dosage inherently have an element of administrative science that might be uncomfortable to some, in spite of the word's Greek root, which means "giving." To those with a more simplistic understanding of modern medicine, dosage also seems to imply a denial of a particularistic, contextual, individualized focus of communication. However, the more modern movement to personalized medicine would seem to encapsulate many of the contemporary trends in communication as well. Medical practitioners know that a therapeutic agent will not work for all people; a good communicologist knows that not all messages will have the same meaning for all people. The science of proteomics promises a new era of personalized medicine where our knowledge of genomics will allow us to much more powerfully predict which agents will work for which people. Historically, cancer research has advanced by determining more and more precisely what is the right amount of poison to administer for specific individuals, depending on the staging of their disease and other factors (Mukherjee, 2010).

There are several key components of a definition of dosage. First, it focuses on an agent that promotes change. Second is the notion that the agent is therapeutic in some sense, that it improves the health and well-being of those who receive it. In a darker way, often a dose needs to be prescribed by an authoritative agent (e.g., doctor) before we can administer it, and it may have unintended or unknown side effects. It also can be associated with agents of infection and with hard luck. Third is the relative amount, duration, and repetition of the agent needed to achieve the desired effect. These factors are known with some precision because of scientific evidence. However, there is one, often hidden difference—communication does not have the underlying science of randomized clinical trials upon which to base its prescriptions.

PLAN OF THE BOOK

This first chapter has provided a framework for applying the basic principles of dosage to the familiar problems of health communicators. In the next chapter we focus on expanding the metaphor of dosage, detailing its many elements as well as discussing the use and limits of metaphor generally.

We then start our focus on contexts by applying the metaphor of dosage to the most elementary of communication contexts—that focusing on relationships between two people in interpersonal communication, especially in terms of their privacy and boundaries. We focus here on physician-patient interactions as an exemplar. Given the complexity of our health care system, increasingly the operation of interdisciplinary teams is critical to health care outcomes, and this will be the focus of our next chapter. Historically mass media theories, such as uses and gratifications, dependency theories, the knowledge gap, as we discuss in chapter 5, have focused on issues of exposure and of resulting media effects. Chapter 6 describes the role of communication in the diffusion and dissemination of scientific advances. Here I also highlight network analysis concepts such as the strength of weak ties, structural equivalence, and social contagion. The most contemporaneously interesting issue of change is the topic addressed in chapter 7. This chapter details the role of communication campaigns and risk communication in these processes.

Chapter 8 focuses on the role of new health information technologies, discussing the impacts of social media, the wisdom of crowds, and the emerging role of m-health. Increasingly researchers exploring new media are discovering that less is often more. So the inundation of people with messages via instant messaging, Twitter, and so on is distracting them from their true tasks rather than informing them of what they should do.

The final chapter turns to broader policy issues raised by application of the metaphor of dosage. It concludes with a discussion of the relationship between researchers and practitioners and how dosage can operate as a bridging metaphor to close the gap between these two traditionally separate roles. Increasingly policy makers, especially in the health field, are resistant to funding research that has no direct practical application.

FURTHER READINGS

Johnson, J. D. (2008). Dosage: A bridging metaphor for theory and practice. *International Journal of Strategic Communication, 2*, 137–153.
  An earlier précis of the dosage metaphor applied to communication.
Lakoff, G., & Johnson, M. (1980). *Metaphors we live by*. Chicago: University of Chicago Press.
  The classic work on metaphors.
Morgan, G. (1986). *Images of organization*. Beverly Hills, CA: Sage.
  A classic of organizational theory that was instrumental in the development of cultural approaches to organization; in-depth treatment of a variety of metaphors commonly used to think about organizations.
Zimmerman, S., Sypher, B. D., & Haas, J. W. (1996). A communication metamyth in the workplace: The assumption that more is better. *Journal of Business Communication, 33*, 185–204.
  Elaboration of the argument of the communication metamyth that more is necessarily better.

Definition and the Use of Metaphor

Human communication will almost always go astray unless real
energy is expended (Reddy, 1979, p. 295)

Metaphors permeate our language, our discourse, and are often fundamental to the ways we think about and act in our social worlds. They have often
been central to how we think about diseases (Mukherjee, 2010; Sontag, 1978,
1988). They are a way of seeing and thinking, providing a way of understanding one thing by appeal to another (Koch & Deetz, 1981), developing a
cognitive bridge between two domains (L. L. Putnam, Phillips, & Chapman,
1996). When using metaphors we apply our knowledge of a familiar subject,
the base domain, to another, the target domain (Grant & Oswick, 1996).
Metaphors can be seen as tools that stimulate us to play with ideas. This playful experimentation is one of the more interesting aspects of metaphor. All
of us, in applying concepts familiar to us to new terrain, are often delighted
with the results, but we are also aware that when we push things too far we
run the risk of degenerating into increasingly silly arguments.

Metaphors also are frequently used by the public at large to communicate. They have become taken-for-granted elements of our everyday lives
and, in this sense, have become "dead" metaphors, since they have become so
commonplace and accepted they are unlikely to result in new insights (Grant
& Oswick, 1996). So, for example, the machine metaphor is commonly used
in descriptions of organizations and is central to *Dilbert* and other satirical
treatments with people viewed as only so many replaceable cogs.

Metaphors can be generative since they may result in new knowledge
about an unfamiliar terrain (Schon, 1979). It is this generative sense that is
the most useful since it can produce new insights by enabling us to see the
world anew, facilitating our understanding of the phenomenon and playful

experimentation with it (Grant & Oswick, 1996). It has become common-place for scholars to apply metaphors to facilitate theory development (Boxenbaum & Rouleau, 2011; Cole & Leide, 2006; Cornelissen, 2006; Morgan, 1986; Oswick, Fleming, & Hanlon, 2011; Palmer & Dunford, 1996), and they have been particularly important in the field of communication (Borisoff & Hahn, 1993; Kalyanaraman & Sundar, 2008; Kaplan, 1990; Krippendorf, 1993; Littlejohn & Foss, 2011; May, 1993; McCorkle & Mills, 1992; J. T. Wood & Phillips, 1980). (See box 2.1 for a discussion of how the dosage

---

BOX 2.1.   COMPARING THE DOSAGE METAPHOR TO CLASSIC COMMUNICATION FORMULATIONS

At this point it would be instructive to directly compare the elements of the dosage metaphor to classic formulations of communication (see table 2.1). One of the very earliest of such formulations was that done by Harold Lasswell (1948), who says what in which channel to whom with what effect. On the dosage side, the first thing one would notice is that the elements of amount, frequency, and sequencing are clearly downplayed in this definition, as they are in most definitions of communication (Dance, 1970). This is especially curious given Lasswell's emphasis on rational, efficient communication in his discussion. Clearly application of the dosage metaphor reemphasizes the importance of variables that are classically associated with the "harder" sciences.

Table 2.1.   Comparing Lasswell's Formulation and the Dosage Metaphor

Lasswell	Dosage Element
Who says	Administrator
What	Therapeutic agent
In which channel	Delivery system
To whom	Recipient
With what effect	Desired outcome

On the other hand, most communication models pay more explicit attention to the "who" and "to whom" elements of the formulation, with more recent work in communication focusing on a dialogic view with a near equal partnership between source and receiver. The consumer movement in health also has resulted in a diminishment of the status differences between the parties in the communication relationship. Lasswell, however, was writing in a much different time, at the beginning of the Cold War, with a near Darwinian attention to the survival of the fittest in contests between nation-states. He clearly saw asymmetrical relationships between the parties in the communication relationship, even going so far as to describe the "who" element in terms of "control analysis." Implicitly in the dosage metaphor there also are clearer status differentials between the parties. Even today in campaign research, which we will return to in much more detail later in this work, there is a heavy emphasis on classic elements of administrative science.

The dosage metaphor takes for granted in many ways the content (what) element of classic communication formulations. In most cases this is viewed as a therapeutic agent that is intended to have one, and only one, effect. In other classic communication models, such as Berlo (1960), there is a recognition that "meanings are in people." The substance that is transmitted is not always the thing that is received, just as genomics realizes that doses are not reacted to in the same way by all patients. Interestingly, however, placebo effects would seem to imply that even for scientifically recognized therapeutic agents, their effect is often determined by how receiver's "interpret" them.

Another way that the dosage metaphor can elaborate on and enrich classic communication formulations is through its emphasis on delivery systems that are key elements of classic pharmaceutical applications, with pronounced differences in impact depending on which method (e.g., intravenous versus oral) is chosen. However, perhaps the most interesting extensions represented by the dosage metaphor come through its notions of interaction and contraindications, as well as the darker side of the dosage metaphor represented in dysfunctional impacts. In some ways desired outcomes are the least interesting results of a dose.

metaphor relates to a classic communication formulation.) The central argument of this book is that dosage is a particularly "live" metaphor, which through its application easily lends itself to richer conceptualizations (Grant & Oswick, 1996) of the role of communication in health.

ELABORATING ON THE DOSAGE METAPHOR

Dosage is derived from a Greek word that literally means the act of giving. In modern usage it is most commonly thought of as the administration of a therapeutic agent in prescribed amounts. Typically these agents are embedded in messages, which can vary in treatment, code, and content, much as drugs can. So the inclusion of metaphors in persuasive messages has been found in a meta-analysis to enhance their impact (Sopory & Dillard, 2002). Classically the media exposure literature has been hampered by the critical mediating factor of attention (Slater, 2004)—whether someone is actually absorbing the dose or whether the body's immune system is actively fighting the dose. This is evocative of Sherif's latitude of rejection notions, which focus on the communication messages that are likely to be persuasive (Sherif & Sherif, 1964). Agents also are impacted by "drug receptors" and differential absorption rates of different organs and notions of absorptive capacity.

We now turn to a more detailed description of the following elements of the dosage metaphor that can enrich our understanding of the work of health professionals: amount, frequency, sequencing, delivery systems, interactions, contraindications, and dysfunctions. We will use these elements to organize our discussion of dosage throughout the remainder of this work.

Amount

> Unlike research on new medications, research on psychosocial treatment rarely considers how much exposure to the intervention is needed to make a difference (Zarit & Femia, 2008, p. 50).

Amount, repetition, and mode of delivery have been central to discussions of exposure and, more generally, media effects (Slater, 2004). But in some ways this is equivalent to the very crude relationships between nutrition and certain health impacts. Foods may contain very healthy individual ingredients and simultaneously contain some very unhealthy ones, as in the case of dark chocolates. Because I like a particular food, I may ingest some elements that are healthy for me, but I do not necessarily do so knowingly. This also may be a very wasteful way of accomplishing a particular end that might be more directly served by taking vitamins.

Frequency

> Life's problems are rarely simple enough to be solved with one dose of not necessarily credible or deep help (Gustafson et al., 2008, p. 254).

Communication theory has generally assumed that repeated messages are more likely to have an impact with direct analogies to medicinal dosages. We don't take one huge dose of a medicine and expect it to last forever. Rather, for the effect to be maintained it needs to be repeated over time. We also may not be able to tolerate huge dosages, but need to gradually accrete certain impacts. But this raises the related issue of the rates of elimination of certain doses, such as recommendations of many campaigns related to cancer screening (e.g., mammography) that are now being revised based on new epidemiological evidence.

Sequencing

The ordering of communication messages, just as the ordering of certain drugs, can produce unique impacts. So I might gradually increase doses of different composition as my tolerance builds. This is somewhat akin to the pathways people follow in acquiring information (J. D. Johnson et al., 2006) since the sequencing of questions may be particularly important for uncertainty reduction (Goldsmith, 2001). Good teachers gradually build students' understanding so they gradually can tolerate more and more in-depth treatments of certain issues.

I might start a search for prevention information with a decision to consult a mediated communication channel (e.g., *Prevention Magazine*), but I also may decide that I want this channel to contain authoritative information as well as a personal touch. This unique hybrid of properties is represented by my health insurance company's telephone hotline. After placing a call I might decide that a particular operator is inexperienced, so I might then decide to try the Web. The website I find in a Google search I evaluate to be more credible, partially because of the nature of the messages it contains. While I can accept the site's message concerning the need for a colonoscopy, I consider the linkage it is suggesting between fat in my diet and colon cancer to be farfetched and discount it. However, we also know that the pathways people follow and whom they are exposed to in their information fields shape their interpretations and determine the answers they obtain and whether or not they obtain them at all. So, Web-based health interventions that tailor information sequentially are often more effective (Sundar et al., 2011), and social marketing often involves a combination of different doses and therapeutic agents (Edgar, Volkman, & Logan, 2011).

Delivery Systems

How a dose is administered can also determine its impact. Some drugs are best taken nasally, whereas others can be taken with a suppository and still others can be taken orally. Similarly communication campaigns often are very strategic in their selection of particular channels, with a well-established maxim that the mass media are best at providing information, while interpersonal channels are often crucial in persuasive efforts. Especially in situations where people are highly motivated, the direct provision of information may be a highly effective strategy (Katz & Kahn, 1978). Alternatively, in the case of certain complex and risky information technologies, direct interpersonal communication and additional training may be necessary ingredients for successful innovation implementation (J. W. Dearing, Meyer, & Kazmierczak, 1994; Fidler & Johnson, 1984).

Interactions

Drugs can have a number of interactions, both positive and negative, as well as contraindications. We are told to take a drug before meals or before bedtime or to not take it with other drugs and to not operate heavy machinery while taking it because of side effects. Similarly, if a source and receiver are homophilous, sharing critical similarities in outlook and perspective, communication is more likely to be effective (Farace, Taylor, & Stewart, 1978).

Contraindications

Pharmacology often rests on the assumption that no drug produces a single effect. There are a number of conditions (e.g., heart problems) in which a particular dose should not be administered. Contraindications are different from interactions, suggesting circumstances for which a dose should definitely not be administered. So a politician whose whole career is based on moral righteousness should never knowingly transmit a duplicitous message. Similarly, violations of private self-disclosures to others can act to permanently damage interpersonal relationships (Petronio & Reierson, 2009).

Dysfunctions

Dosage also has a darker side. People can become too dependent on particular therapeutic agents, leading to problems with withdrawal, addiction, and various forms of substance abuse. They also can believe more is necessarily better, leading to problems with overdosage and continuation long after any benefit has occurred. Increasing attention is also being given to the nocebo effect, where patients experienced negative side effects to a drug because they expected to, which is especially evident in chemotherapy (Cloud, 2009).

These problems, in turn, can lead to resistance to the beneficial effects of therapeutic agents when they are truly needed, much like what has occurred with antibiotics and their overusage in the United States. At times, the wrong drug, such as high-powered antibiotics, can treat the symptoms but not the underlying cause of the disease. We have also seen in very competitive situations people who risk substantial long-term issues with their health to inject themselves with performance-enhancing drugs of various sorts.

In intrapersonal communication frequent mulling about conflicts leads to people feeling worse and worse without increasing understanding of the conflict; however, this can be ameliorated by more frequent, direct interpersonal communication with the other (Cloven & Roloff, 1991). Metaphors dealing with interpersonal conflict are often dominated by the dark side (e.g., war, conquest, and so on), often making their resolution more difficult

(McCorkle & Mills, 1992). Similarly, other metaphors, such as the student as consumer, have the unfortunate consequence of commodifying education and increasing the distance between administrators, faculty, and students (McMillan & Cheney, 1996).

THE LIMITS OF METAPHOR

> Seen as allegories or as figures of speech, metaphors may appear to be no more than simple literary or linguistic tools, yet there is far more to them than that. They are the outcome of the cognitive process that is in constant use—a process in which the literal meaning of the phrase or word is applied to the content in a figurative sense (Grant & Oswick, 1996, p. 1).

Metaphors are so pervasive and elemental to human thought that some see the use of metaphors as inevitable (Grant & Oswick, 1996). As with any tool, however, a practitioner needs to be aware of its limitations and whether another tool might be more appropriate. The central issue of this work is, Does the metaphor of dosage help us to understand the role of health communicators? In this section I will discuss some of the limitations of metaphor.

With roots tracing back to Aristotle, metaphor and comparison have been traditional tools of the communication discipline (Cornelissen, 2005). However, there has been some controversy over the extent to which the application of metaphor can truly move beyond comparison and correspondence (Oswick & Jones, 2006) to a more creative, emergent, near dialogic view (Cornelissen, 2005, 2006). Dialogue is becoming an increasing feature of the world of health professionals, both with other professionals and also with patients whose worlds are often premised on different views than our own. Dialogue, feedback from application of metaphor, and resulting anomalous comparisons can extend our understanding of both the metaphor and the situation to which it is applied (Cornelissen, 2005).

The ultimate hope in the development of any metaphor is to specify potential new lines for theory and for empirical research (Cornelissen, 2005; Palmer & Dunford, 1996). At its most heuristic a metaphor must involve objects of comparison that are at some distance from each other to offer unique and meaningful insights, emanating in part from surprise (Cornelissen, 2006). But the degree of distance is also a source of tension because of potentially inherent residual dissimilarities (Cornelissen, 2005).

The value of a metaphor is often in the eye of the beholder. Some can question its application in one or more particulars. So, some might question whether the simplest vision of the dosage metaphor, taking a pill, really applies to the richness of communication. However, the emerging science of proteomics suggests that things are much more complex, that some medicines work best when we have detailed knowledge of the genetic receptivity of the "audience." Similarly, major theories of attitude change contrast the mindful rather than passive processing of messages as important for their ultimate efficacy.

Metaphors may also seriously mislead us in understanding the phenomenon to which they are applied (Grant & Oswick, 1996), often through their latent entailments (Krippendorf, 1993). We must be careful. The conduit metaphor when applied to communication often implies that the content of messages can easily flow along constrained pathways from a source to receiver without loss of intended meanings. The most fundamental latent assumption in the dosage metaphor relates to the often taken-for-granted assumption that there is a cure for any problem. Metaphors may serve to reify latent ideological positions and may serve as an inertial force that protects us from critical inspection that can lead to mindful reforms (Grant & Oswick, 1996).

While metaphors can be liberating, one of their major limitations for members of social groups is their exclusionary potential. They can privilege certain groups. Those who have participated in team sports may have greater facility with the use of associated metaphors in the emerging contemporary world of interprofessional teams. For the dosage metaphor, those with a medical background and a more functionalist, administrative bent may be privileged.

CONCLUSION

It has been argued that people cannot think about communication without appealing to metaphor (Krippendorf, 1993) and that metaphors provide an "imaginative rationality" (Lakoff & Johnson, 1980, p. 193). Perhaps the most controversial aspect of the application of metaphors stems from their often very playful nature and the resulting messiness (Grant & Oswick, 1996). Scientists can view metaphors as antithetical to the scientific enterprise since they are not easily quantified. In some ways, then, uses of the dosage metaphor may be particularly ironic since fundamentally dosage deals with quantity. Metaphors cannot be easily measured; nor can their fit to a particular problem be precisely quantified as in a statistical test. Fundamentally metaphors are in the eyes of the beholder: either they are useful, or they are not.

FURTHER READINGS

Dance, F. E. X. (1970). The "concept" of communication. *Journal of Communication, 20*, 201–210.

A systematic review of definitions of communication isolates 15 main themes (e.g., understanding, transfer). Dance suggests that there are three main dimensions along which definitions can be split: level of observation, intent, and normative judgment.

Reddy, M. J. (1979). The conduit metaphor—a case of frame conflict in our language about language. In A. Ortony (Ed.), *Metaphor and thought* (pp. 284–324). Cambridge: Cambridge University Press.

Provides numerous examples of how the conduit metaphor permeates everyday language about communication; for example, "let me know if you *find* any good *ideas* in the *essay*" (p. 288, italics in original). Reddy goes on to argue that this common view suggests communication is relatively effortless for the sender, with most of the responsibility for successful communication resting on the receiver to successfully put the right message into the words that will be delivered.

• 3 •

Interpersonal Communication

$\mathscr{A}$t its most elemental level interpersonal communication refers to the context in which two people are interacting with each other. Often interpersonal communication dwells on issues that directly relate to the dosage metaphor, including work relating to the question of intimacy and boundaries, which focuses on how much I reveal to the other, which some view as central to truly interpersonal communication. Physician-patient interactions are a very rich context for examining these issues, in part because, while they are face-to-face, they often do not meet the expectations patients have in truly interpersonal encounters, and they can be used as an exemplar of a variety of relationships between various health professionals and clients. It is important that the messages that a patient receives during all of these encounters be consonant since repetition of the same message from a variety of sources is often a key to understanding (Bottorff et al., 1998). (See box 3.1 for an example.)

Interpersonal theories explore commonly used metaphors (e.g., the depths of a relationship, dominance themes, exchange, boundaries, containers, fairy tales). The source metaphor of journey has often been used to describe the end point of a course of treatment. So you have the physician as guide; the events in the relationship; the progress made, expressed as the distance covered (and perhaps the number of different places visited, associated with wisdom); the overcoming of obstacles; forks in the road, describing the choices at different points of therapy; the duration of the relationship; and ultimately the final destination.

BOX 3.1.   INFORMATION PRESCRIPTIONS

While there has been much concern over patients/clients use of the Internet in the search for information, given the often problematic quality of the information they find, which we will discuss in more detail in the chapter on health information technology, until recently there have not been proactive efforts to guide their searches. There would seem to be a substantial advantage for health information services to operate in concert with physicians in this endeavor (J. D. Johnson, 2005). They could, in effect, arrange their services to provide more detailed information for those who would like it and to insure that the information services that patients use are of high quality.

These concerns have been most recently expressed in systematic attempts to provide information prescriptions to patients. Just as patients get prescriptions for drugs, they would get written prescriptions for websites to consult related to their medical problems. This concept has been embraced by the National Library of Medicine in their Medline Plus website. They have partnered with the American College of Physicians Foundation to assist physicians in this endeavor, developing an Information Rx Tool Kit to assist clinicians in developing appropriate materials.

Research trials of this idea have found that it increases use of authoritative sites such as Medline Plus and that patients were more likely to find this information valuable if their physician prescribed it. The physicians involved in these trials found that there was greater patient compliance and reduced office time spent on education and that they helped to explain difficult concepts (Coberly et al., 2010).

PHYSICIAN-PATIENT RELATIONSHIPS

The physician-patient relationship is obviously one of great pragmatic importance, especially with our attention turned to the funding of our health care system (Epstein & Street, 2007). There are six core functions in the patient-clinician communication relationship: fostering healing relationships, exchanging information, responding to emotions, managing uncertainty, making decisions, and enabling patient self-management (Epstein & Street, 2007). The accomplishment of all these functions is heavily dependent on dosage-related issues. In this connection, interestingly, "thin slices" of behavior such as tone of voice or a grimace, as is also the case in the development of first impressions generally, can lead to global judgments of the respect for and trust in physicians and outcomes such as greater likelihood of malpractice suits (Roter & Hall, 2011).

Historically these relationships have been viewed from a deficit model with a focus on insufficient information as a result of lack of its provision by clinicians (Epstein & Street, 2007). More recent approaches have focused on a process model where a clinician monitors the amount of information being provided to patients and helps them interpret it so that they do not become overloaded and can truly participate in decision making (Epstein & Street, 2007). This focus on the process model directly relates to a paradox: "the same communication behaviors may improve some outcomes, but worsen others" (Epstein & Street, 2007, p. 42). So, while providing information can act to relieve anxiety and uncertainty in one area, it also may act to heighten concerns in others. Thus, a definitive diagnosis of cancer can reduce uncertainty, but it raises a whole host of other concerns. Some have suggested that for terminally ill patients, communicating with metaphors offers a more sensitive means of communicating bad news (Hutchings, 1998).

A persistent puzzle has been a large percentage of patients who don't comply with medical prescriptions or with other doctor's instructions, with estimates ranging from 50% to 30%, respectively, for these two aspects of medical care historically (Lane, 1983). (For more detail see box 3.2.) More recently, a World Health Organization (2003) study found only 50% of patients with chronic diseases in developed countries were in concordance with treatment recommendations. For one specific class of drugs, statins, patients were at 50% adherence at six months and 30% to 40% within one year (Bandolier, 2004). Chronic disease patients often stop taking medicines within 30 days of their treatments' onset (Kreps, 2009). It has been estimated that noncompliant patients nearly double treatment time and the complications that they have and that the cost of their care is four times that of compliant ones (Lane, 1983).

However, in spite of considerable research attention, a magic bullet still hasn't been found to achieve higher levels of adherence (Kreps, 2009). This is in part because compliance is almost exclusively defined in terms of the perspective of medical providers, who often explicitly and implicitly blame patients for being uncooperative (Lane, 1983). It appears that noncompliance does not vary with the severity of illness, duration of disease, and so on. The one variable that does appear to affect compliance directly is the complexity of potential treatments (Lane, 1983). In chapter 7, we will note that complexity puts an absolute limit on the amount of communication necessary for the implementation of innovations. This directly relates to another positive contributor to compliance, that is, doctors providing education, often repeatedly, to their patients about important aspects of their illness and treatment (Brown, Stewart, & Ryan, 2003; Lane, 1983).

One of the many interesting paradoxical findings in this literature is a potential dose-response relationship between information about personalized

---

BOX 3.2.   COMPLIANCE GAINING

Often the most critical outcomes of a physician-patent interaction is compliance with a recommended course of treatment. Put simply, compliance gaining represents attempts to get the other to do what you want. This is done for a variety of reasons, some of them altruistic. One of the key issues in compliance gaining research involves the use of power: what amounts and types are necessary to achieve particular purposes. A key assumption of this approach is that of match—the idea that you select particular tactics and strategies to fit a situation and your desired outcomes. This area of research has received considerable attention in interpersonal communication focusing often on typologies of compliance gaining strategies based on the seminal early work of Marwell and Schmitt (1967) and is heavily concerned with intentional, strategic approaches to interpersonal communication.

As an example, let us trace the different strategies an internist might use in treating high blood pressure. She might start with *showing expertise about negative outcomes*, detailing such bad things that might happen if it is not controlled as kidney failure. Before doing this she might indicate *liking* for the patient, indicating her concern for them as a person, and detailing *moral appeals* by indicating the patient's responsibility to their children and spouse. She also may imply family members will *show positive* esteem to the patient as a result of their compliance. She might sketch some *negative altercasting*, suggesting only the most slothful and irresponsible of her patients do not control their blood pressure. In a way, these strategies reflect amount and treatment issues associated with dosage, so if one strategy appears not to be working, one should switch to another strategy. There is also the possibility that some may backfire, resulting in dysfunctional consequences.

These strategies can be employed to achieve compliance, manipulate consequences, improve one's relational position, or define values and obligations (Littlejohn & Foss, 2011). One interesting controversy within the compliance gaining literature is, When does one have the right to persuade (Littlejohn, 1992)? This right is taken for granted in the context of physician-patient relationships. It is generally recognized that the use of compliance gaining strategies is important for doctor-patient relationships, since a major part of medical practice relates to persuading patients to engage in positive health-related activities.

---

risk and intention to engage in cancer screening. It appears that the more detailed the communication about such risk, the less patients feel the need to participate in screening since they often relate this to a marginal personal gain from the activity (Epstein & Street, 2007). While there is some evidence that longer visits are associated with more negative outcomes, education often takes considerable time, and in our cost-driven health care system, this time often is not available (Brown, Stewart, & Ryan, 2003). Longer visits encourage patients to express concerns and receive answers (Real & Street, 2009). Under capitation HMO plans, the physician's mantra can become "Do less, earn more," which translates into "Communicate less, earn more" (Brown, Stewart, & Ryan, 2003). One way of coping with this issue is the use of medical decision support systems described in box 3.3.

BOX 3.3.   MEDICAL DECISION SUPPORT SYSTEMS

A variety of software systems exist to aid decision-making processes. They often focus on access to databases and other types of information that can facilitate this work. These systems have existed for decades, and several systems have been commercialized, but they have not often fulfilled the hype devoted to them (Power, 2007).

In medicine these systems have been used to facilitate the decision making of patients, physicians, and other health professionals. They do this by leading the decision maker step-by-step through often complicated decision trees. More advanced systems can take on a gamelike feel and are linked to authoritative evidence. In clinical work these systems are often used to reduce medical errors by decreasing reliance on memory and increasing access to evidence-based medicine. These systems provide alerts and reminders, diagnostic assistance, therapy critiquing and planning, prescribing information, image recognition, and interpretation guidance (Coiera, 2003). While they often improve practitioner performance, a systematic review has found only inconsistent evidence that they improve patient outcomes (Garg et al., 2005).

Algorithms constituting an inference engine to facilitate clinical decision making are often embedded in electronic medical records, where they often rest on evidence-based practice and are used as diagnostic aids (Coiera, 2003). However, their use has been criticized by physicians as being as much of a hindrance as a facilitator to clinical judgment (Groopman, 2007; Sweeney, 2006). They also can require more time and effort than traditional methods (Coiera, 2003; Garg et al., 2005).

Their proponents make very strong claims about the improved decision making that results from these rather expensive systems (Hoffman, 1994). Unfortunately these claims have yet to be supported in research studies, in part because organizations modify these systems in use to reflect their cultures. Clinical decision support systems are often "homegrown" products of local champions; as a result, they have limited exportability and problematic updates to new enterprise systems and other upgrades (Garg et al., 2005). There are literally hundreds of systems that have been developed, which creates problems in sharing data (Raghavan, 2005). However, in actual use they may also be limited in the same way that other processes are—by the limits of human decision making and the artificial boundaries imposed upon them by a system's culture (Poole & DeSanctis, 1992).

Unfortunately, little attention is devoted in physician training to the appropriate means of achieving compliance among their patients to recommended treatments (Gillotti, 2003; Lane, 1983). Needless to say, this is particularly unfortunate because this is where "the rubber meets the road"; without this critical last step, often very sophisticated medical treatments are for naught. Physicians who show more empathy and spend more time with a patient are more likely to be the sole source of information and ultimately achieve greater compliance (Tustin, 2010). Estimates of noncompliance range from 25% to 40% for certain chronic diseases like diabetes, with noncompliance linked to a lack of concordance between physician and patient in goals, understanding of medical condition (Haskard, Williams, & DiMatteo, 2009), and vocabulary. In effect, physicians have little understanding of the dosage needed in communication terms to achieve appropriate outcomes, partly because of the lack of research in this area, which has resulted in few guidelines for them (Epstein & Street, 2007). The basic problem for these relationships is that neither party truly understands the other's goals (Epstein & Street, 2007). Physicians who match the preferences of their patients are more likely to have satisfied patients who are less likely to pursue malpractice suits (Duggan & Thompson, 2011).

In the absence of considerable progress on the physician side, more and more attention, especially given our recent focus on patients as consumers, has been devoted to issues of patient self-advocacy and the active role that they can play in health care decision making (Epstein & Street, 2007; Wright, Frey, & Sopory, 2007). Patients who are more assertive in their information seeking are more likely to receive answers that allow them to make informed health care decisions (Real & Street, 2009). However, even the most dedicated patient can quickly become overloaded with the amount of information available through the Internet and other sources (Epstein & Street, 2007). This is but one indication of the importance of contextual factors in this dyadic relationship. Especially important is the time that doctors have with patients (Real & Street, 2009) to deliver the appropriate communication dose.

RELATIONSHIPS AS EXCHANGES

Notions of exchange have been a central theoretical starting point to many interpersonal communication theories. For example, equity in emotional exchanges has been seen as a cornerstone of relational maintenance (Stafford, 2005; Stafford & Canary, 1991). In this view individuals are seen as driven to maximize rewards through their interaction with each other. Exchange relationships are often embedded in the more encompassing metaphor of markets, which often have somewhat of a negative connotation in interpersonal contexts (e.g., meat markets for initial dating encounters). Markets operate to diffuse information rapidly to interested parties (F. von Hayek, 1991) in an overall configuration often cast as traders in a bazaar (Geertz, 1973, 1978). A focus on exchanges provides a theoretic focus for the development of relationships between people, who may otherwise lack compelling motives to interact. We often seek exchanges with others precisely because they are not like us, and they have resources that we do not possess.

The nature of relationships in markets often rests on achieving a fair price for a good or service. In pure market exchange relationships the only thing that may matter is the value of the goods exchanged. Normative controls may also be operative (Lorenz, 1991; Powell, 1990), and the consequences of untrustworthy behavior may hamper the further development of relationships (Kirman, 2001). These issues make the importance of openness, self-disclosure, and privacy even more telling.

HOW MUCH DO I REVEAL? WHEN?

One of the fundamental issues in everyday interpersonal communication relates to how open one is with the other and the degree of self-disclosure one engages in (which often rests on equal exchanges). In fact many view this issue to be central to definitions of interpersonal communication. It is also wrapped up in notions of privacy and boundaries in relationships. However, in the typical physician-patient interaction there is a lack of reciprocation, and these relationships are very one-sided. This may cause some inherent difficulties in these relationships, since normally when people reveal their deepest, most private concerns, they expect the other to provide them with something of equal value in exchange.

Openness

> In fact there is abundant evidence that long-term relationships
> are maintained by illusions of truth, exaggerations of goodness
> . . . and less than full communication (Bochner, 1982, p. 120).

In self-disclosure information about oneself is purposively communicated to the other. It can differ in depth and breadth, which determine the degree of intimacy in a relationship. A physician-patient interaction depends on one-sided self-disclosure, which unfortunately all too often does not happen. People are often very reluctant to share totally with a physician their concerns, especially if there is a stigma attached to them.

Self-disclosure research historically had its roots in humanistic psychology and the ideology of honest communication (Parks, 1982) with a cultural myth, suggesting that increased openness is helpful for relationships (Stafford, 2003; Stafford & Canary, 1991), a view that has been increasingly questioned (Afifi & Afifi, 2009). It asserts that interpersonal and personal understanding occurs through self-disclosure, feedback, and sensitivity to others. In this view the ideal interpersonal relationship is one in which both parties fully and openly experience each other, which health professionals are often reluctant to do since it may reveal to clients their own doubts and reservations, ultimately diminishing their professional standing.

Research in this area started with the hypothesis that disclosure leads to liking, attraction, and positive perceptions of the other's character. This type of communication permits the continued growth of the individual. And the intimacy of relationships between the parties increases if communication is of this particular kind (Littlejohn, 1989). Generally four dimensions of this concept have been identified, all with parallels to the dosage metaphor: breadth, or the number of topics; depth, or the intimacy of the content; duration; and valence, whether the disclosure is positive or negative (Bochner, 1982). Certainly a physician-patient interaction often limits at least two of these dimensions: breadth and duration.

There also are clear norms as to the amount of reciprocity suggesting that if one shares a certain amount and kind with you, you need to reciprocate. Further, it is suggested that the reduced likelihood that the other will share information disclosed to them by the other outside the dyad results in greater disclosure (Parks, 1982). Somewhat akin to a dosage metaphor, there also needs to be a recognition of the time and energy that a truly intimate relationship involves (Parks, 1982).

Bochner (1982) has argued a second vision, Vision II, of interpersonal communication that emerged with the counterculture of the 1960s and 1970s. Self-disclosure became the expression of private feelings, thoughts, and characteristics. Bochner (1984) has pointed out that inappropriate self-disclosures can actually produce negative impressions, and people may be reluctant to self-disclose for fear it might damage their relationships, indicating a sensitivity to side effects for this "therapeutic agent." So, alcoholics, drug addicts, and others who have ailments with stigma attached may be reluctant to self-disclose. Research in this area has resulted in a growing appreciation for the many dysfunctional aspects of self-disclosure and circumstances where it is contraindicated. Also, research findings have indicated very highly disclosive individuals are judged to be less intelligent, less well adjusted, and less likable (Parks, 1982). Doctors too may run into the too-much-information problem.

There are many potential benefits to self-disclosure, including catharsis, maintenance of positive relationships, validating self-concepts, bringing a sense of cohesion, fulfilling ethical obligations, achieving greater social influence, securing social support, and so on. But it also can have many dysfunctional consequences, including potential loss of relationship depending on content reaction of others, loss of self-concept and esteem, privacy violations on the part of the other, loss of influence and face, infliction of harm on the other, and so on.

Sometimes people feel freer to be more intimate with strangers with whom they do not share a social context, since there are fewer potential negative consequences, than with close acquaintances and friends. It also has been suggested that openness plays a more equivocal role in relational maintenance, with findings suggesting an inversely negative relationship after controlling for such factors as positivity (Stafford, 2003). Accordingly, by and large the initially optimistic vision has been replaced by a more strategic one that suggests that the disclosure of information be selective, focusing on positive contents. Interestingly, married partners engage in less openness than those engaged or seriously dating. Only a very small percentage of communication with others, even our intimates, contains the level of self-disclosure that the early literature in this area suggested. This realization has resulted in a renewed interest in privacy and boundaries. At times, in some institutional settings like university hospitals, patients may be reluctant to reveal things, even with HIPAA protections, because it may be too risky if they became common knowledge.

Privacy

Sandra Petronio (2002) has been engaged in a systematic research program focusing on the boundaries of privacy. She is grappling with the question of whether or not to tell, with a subsidiary issue of how much to reveal, something patients routinely struggle with in office visits. Since people want to feel that they are the rightful owners of their personal information, and since there are risks to disclosure (e.g., disclosing at a bad time, telling too much about ourselves), people want to control how much information they give to the other, engaging in conscious risk assessments concerning self-disclosure. But there are also potential payoffs to disclosing private information to others, especially in terms of enhanced intimacy. Once information is shared, it becomes co-owned, with negotiated rights and responsibilities for both parties.

Petronio's (2002) Communication Privacy Management (CPM) theory consciously uses the metaphor of boundaries to illustrate the flow of private information to others. Five basic suppositions underlie its rule management system. First, the focus is on private information. Second, the boundary metaphor illustrates the demarcation between private information and public relationships. Third, concealing private information makes one feel vulnerable, and relatedly people believe that private information is owned or co-owned by others. Fourth, decisions about boundary regulation are based on the rule management system. Fifth, privacy and disclosure are dialectic forces in relationships.

CPM suggests that not all disclosures of private information result in intimacy. Many other factors are at play, one of which is frequency, which directly evokes an element of dosage. Once information is disclosed and thus "co-owned" by the other, a resulting breach of confidentiality may be one of the few situations where one dose, without repetition, can have lasting impacts (Petronio & Reierson, 2009). Physicians are often legally compelled to share certain private information, like gunshot wounds, infectious diseases, and so on, leading patients who know this to be less likely to seek medical treatment.

Social Penetration Theory

> A relationship undergoing the process of deterioration should move from *more* to *less* intimate and from *greater* to *lesser* amounts of interaction—contrary to the forward penetration process (Altman & Taylor, 1973, p. 7, italics in original).

Self-disclosure is central to Altman and Taylor's Social Penetration Theory (Altman & Taylor, 1973). They suggest social penetration gradually progresses during a relationship from superficial nonintimate areas to more intimate central areas. This is often the result of reciprocal giving of information, which often is not present in inherently one-sided relationships involving health care providers.

Greater depth and breadth of self-disclosures can determine the nature of relationships. Breadth frequency is determined by the number of different topical areas, or breadth categories, open to another person and the amount of interaction in each of them. As we have seen, often there is very little breadth in the typically biomedically driven physician-patient encounter. Similarly to exchange processes, rewards and costs often drive social penetration within a relationship. More modern views suggest relational avoidance, perhaps associated with the too-much-information problem, results from a direct linear function of relational closeness (Afifi & Afifi, 2009).

Altman and Taylor suggest there are four stages to a relationship, which echoes the dosage element of sequencing. The orientation stage is characterized by stereotypes and superficial knowledge of the other. The exploratory affective exchange stage is characterized by initial attempts at self-disclosure that one desires to be reciprocated. Affective exchange deals with deeper, more intimate areas central to the personality. Finally, during the stable exchange stage, people fully understand each other, and communication is more efficient.

SUMMARY AND COMMENTARY

One of the most compelling sets of research findings in the social science literature in the last couple of decades relates to the relative social isolation of Americans. Robert Putnam (2000) detailed in his book *Bowling Alone* the decline in membership in social groupings and the impacts this has on a larger sense of community. Similarly, a series of network analysis studies have detailed that, on average, Americans have very few people whom they can share personal information with. In 1985 the General Social Survey asked a nationally representative sample of Americans how many confidants they had with whom they could discuss important matters. This survey was followed up in 2004, with depressing results: the number of people saying there was no one nearly tripled. The mean network size decreased by about a third from around three in 1985 to around two in 2004. There were dramatic decreases in nonkin ties and fewer contacts in voluntary associations and neighborhoods. There also appears to be a pronounced tendency to have contacts with others like oneself (McPherson, Smith-Lovin, & Brashears, 2006). All of this suggests that the sort of intimate, disclosive relationships that have historically been the "gold standard" of interpersonal communication are very much the exception, not the rule.

In the interpersonal communication literature there has been a growing recognition that our separate relationships are affected by the relationships we have with others (Milardo, 1983). Thus our dyadic relationships are seen as affected by their embeddedness in social contexts, such as the interprofessional teams we turn to in the next chapter. The work of Parks and his colleagues has been particularly important in this regard (Parks & Adelman, 1983; Parks, Stan, & Eggert, 1983). For example, Eggert and Parks (1987) found general support for hypotheses connecting relational development factors (e.g., sociability, intimacy, and commitment) and communication network factors among adolescents. Dyadic relationships are increasingly being seen as embedded in the larger macro contexts of organizations from cultural, climate, or system perspectives.

The amount of self-disclosure is generally considered to be an important indication of the intimacy of a relationship. Discordant interpersonal relationships often stem from a lack of match between the degree of self-disclosure within a relationship and what both parties perceive as the stage of the relationship. Lack of trust in a partner may contraindicate a tendency to self-disclose. Classically there also is a key reciprocal component to self-disclosure. When one discloses something about oneself, it is expected that the other will also disclose similarly intimate topics.

Self-disclosure appears to be another example of curvilinear impacts and match issues that are directly related to the dosage metaphor. Similar dynamics are present in compliance gaining research in terms of the match of appropriate strategies to outcomes desired (see table 3.1).

Table 3.1.   Comparing Interpersonal Approaches and the Dosage Metaphor

	Interpersonal Approaches	
Dosage Elements	*Boundaries (Openness, Privacy)*	*Compliance Gaining*
Amount	Threshold, how much to reveal	Goal dependent
Frequency	One time	Goal dependent
Sequencing	Progressive, reciprocal, timing critical	Strategic
Delivery systems	Face-to-face assumed for intimacy	Interpersonal primary, other channels complement
Interactions	Trust	Social milieu
Contraindications	Disclosure could damage	Outside influences
Dysfunctions	Ideology of openness	Paternalistic, one-way, ethical concerns

Frequency is dealt with differently in interpersonal approaches. One critical self-disclosure or negative relational comment can have lasting impacts on a relationship. The frequency of various compliance gaining strategies is determined by the outcomes associated with them. Sequencing often comes to the fore in the increasing intimacy often assumed as a natural progression of relationships. So there is a presumption of successively more intimate disclosures. The notions of over- and underbenefiting and inequity driving relationships also suggest a degree of reciprocity and follow-on expectation in relationships driven by exchange dynamics. The use of compliance gaining strategies in physician-patient relationships is often determined by the severity of diagnosis and prognosis. Interpersonal approaches are the most reductionist and most limited in what they have to say about delivery systems, although some work on physician-patient interactions suggests they should be supplemented by other media, such as brochures and surfing the Internet.

There are critical interactive factors in each of the major approaches we have discussed in the section: trust is critical to self-disclosure, distance is critical to strategies used in long-distance relationships, and the social milieu one is in affects compliance gaining strategies that are used. Similarly, there are clear contraindications: disclosure is limited if it is perceived that it could damage the relationship or that someone might reveal private information to others.

Areas of dysfunctions have also been revealed in this chapter. First, the ideology of openness may have caused significant harm to relationships. Second, compliance gaining strategies in physician-patient relationships often result in an overly paternalistic, one-way approach to these relationships that may impact a patient's adherence to treatment protocols, and reactions to genetic information are critical to personalized media, as detailed in box 3.4.

BOX 3.4.   GENETIC TESTING

The marketing of genetic testing to the general population . . . could act to induce demand for these services in
a health care system that is currently unequipped to meet
this demand. Education remains a vital tool in addressing
the concerns of those patients requesting genetic testing
from their health care provider (Bunn et al. 2002, p. 576).

We have learned that cancer is, at its core, the consequence
of alterations in DNA—that cancer is a genetic disease.
Genetic information has the potential to transform how
we prevent, detect, and treat cancer (Klausner, 1996, p. 36).

While rapid advances in genetics research promise enhanced care, the inherent
complexities and individualistic nature of genetic information have resulted in a
challenging information environment. The technical possibilities for acquiring
genomic information are increasing at an exponential pace, as are the scientific
advances relating to it. Furthermore, societal reactions to genomics and possible privacy and discrimination issues may constitute significant constraints.
The health care infrastructure also has its limits, given the severe shortage of
qualified genetic counselors and general practitioners who are unprepared to
address genetics, creating a demand for creative approaches to service delivery.

A variety of studies have found that people are less likely to look for information as their distance from cancer decreases (Helmes et al., 2000). For example,
Degner and Sloan (1992) found that while 64% of the general public felt they
would want to select their own treatment if they had cancer, 59% of patients
wanted physicians to make these decisions on their behalf. Similarly, Armstrong
et al. (2002) found that interest in testing was inversely related to a family history
of breast cancer. Interestingly, inclusion of risk information in direct-to-consumer
websites actually decrease intention of test for BRCA (S. W. Gray et al., 2009).

Genetic information, particularly related to testing, screening, and personalized medicine, poses some unique challenges for individuals; it also can
have potentially negative social (e.g., insurance coverage, discrimination),
financial (e.g., costs of testing), and psychological consequences (Armstrong,
Schwartz, & FitzGerald, 2002; Kelly et al., 2007; Rothstein, 1997). Yet there
are potentially significant health benefits for individuals who can achieve efficacious access to and use of pertinent information (F. S. Collins et al., 2003).
Not only will people have precise information about their relative risks, which
could result in more focused prevention behaviors, but treatments could be
specifically targeted based on one's genetic makeup. However, there are many
perils in the ever-growing area of direct-to-consumer genetic testing: lack of

continued

BOX 3.4.   *Continued*

clinical validity of some tests, overutilization in low-risk individuals, uncertain quality of tests, inadequate counseling, and misinterpretation of results (S. W. Gray et al., 2009). Genomics also has the potential to become an ideology that places increasing burdens and responsibilities on individuals, which contributes to the culture of surveillance of the worried well and the perception that everyone is sick or potentially so (Silva, 2005).

The US public is interested in issues surrounding genetics and genetic testing, and they are aware these advances may affect their health care decisions (Andrews et al., 2005; F. S. Collins et al., 2003). This also relates to the general interest in genealogies and family medical histories (D. O. Case, 2008). In a national survey more than a third of adults said they had closely followed the developments leading to the mapping of the human genome, and nearly two-thirds of the respondents felt that they were likely to take a genetic test if it could identify whether they were at risk of contracting a disease (Avins, 2000a). Other studies in the scientific literature support these general findings. For instance, a general population survey found high levels of interest in genetic testing (82%) (Andrykowski et al., 1997). Regarding cancer genetics in particular, Andrykowski, Munn & Studts (1996) again found high interest in predictive genetic testing for cancer in general (87%) and breast cancer in particular (93%).

Reactions to information regarding the many diseases that may be inherited through the human genome varies (Jallinoja et al., 1998). While it is estimated that only 5% to 10% of cancers may be genetically determined (Bell, 1998; Bottorff et al., 1998; Kash et al., 2000; Sidransky, 1996; Stopfer, 2000), the public generally is unaware of the basics of genetics (Bottorff et al., 1998; Croyle & Lerman, 1999) and has been found to vastly overestimate their individual risks (Bottorff et al., 1998; Croyle & Lerman, 1999; Kash et al., 2000). For example, Bluman et al. (1999) found 60% of women with breast cancer and/or ovarian cancer overestimated their risk. "Interest in undergoing testing is more strongly related to perceived risk than objective risk" (Marteau & Croyle, 1998, p. 695); so the demand for information related to genetics is likely to be great even among women who are not likely to have predisposing mutations (Kash et al., 2000; Lerman, et al., 1995; Ludman et al., 1999). For low-risk individuals, however, brief counseling can result in substantial benefits in lowering anxiety (Stopfer, 2000) and the high levels of worry in the general public (Durfy et al., 1999). In fact, Lerman et al. (1999) revealed that about half of their interviewees indicated that negative test results would lead to unhealthy behavior, possibly due to either false reassurance or a misunderstanding of risk. Indeed, determining that someone may have a genetic predisposition may trigger a stream of questions that, at least for a while, may actually increase the uncertainty of individuals (Sherer & Juanillo, 1992). Policy makers are also increasingly concerned with the psychological stress that results from false-positive results that are a substantial disadvantage of cancer screening (Wardle et al., 1993).

Thus, mirroring classic findings in the attitude literature, which find relatively low correlations among knowledge, attitudes, and behavior (Bettinghaus, 1986), there is a significant decline in the proportions of individuals who express the same desire when confronted with the possibility that they may actually have cancer (Bilodeau & Degner, 1996). Lerman et al. (1996) showed actual uptake of genetic testing within an at-risk population for hereditary breast-ovarian cancer was lower than anticipated from previous studies, with only 43% of all study subjects requesting test results. Welkenhuysen et al. (2001) also found that women with breast cancer relatives were much less interested in a predictive test than those without them. Armstrong et al. (2002) found that family history of breast cancer was *inversely* related to interest in genetic testing, something also found in Kentucky (Andrykowski et al., 1997). Helmes et al. (2000) demonstrated that while many women were initially interested in a study of genetic counseling for breast cancer, "higher cancer worry scores meant less likelihood of participation in the study" (p. 1379). In spite of prior studies that indicated 83% of the general population and 82% of first-degree relatives of colon cancer patients were interested in receiving a genetic test, Lerman et al. (1999) found that only 43% of adults in extended HNPCC families chose to receive the results of tests they had taken.

The decline in intent levels is directly linked to perceptions of the disease, with only 10% of clients seeking genetic tests when there is no efficacious treatment and/or it is fatal, 50% seeking testing for breast cancer for which there is hope for both treatment and prevention, and 80% seeking treatment for diseases with effective treatments (Marteau & Croyle, 1998). So, 13% of adults tested for HIV never received results (a figure that nearly doubled for those whose tests were not self-initiated) (Hurley, Kosenko & Brashers, 2011). For Huntington's chorea, a particularly devastating genetic disease with no effective treatment, in principle, two-thirds of persons at risk expressed an interest in testing, while only 15% actually came forward to be tested when the test was available (Lerman et al., 1995), and similar results were found a decade later (Wahlin, 2007). People at risk for a severe, untreatable disease tended to decline a genetic test and did not even want to read about it privately (Dawson, Savitsky, & Dunning, 2006).

A decline in interest in testing is also associated with accurate assessments of genetic risk factors, with a greater understanding of the limitations and uncertainties surrounding testing, with concerns over confidentiality and insurance, and so on (Geller et al., 1995). In addition, psychological processes related to denial may also have an impact. For example, of the 26% of the sample who said they would be very or somewhat unlikely to take a test, 41% said they would rather not know if they were at risk of disease (Avins, 2000b). This overall pattern of findings raises significant policy questions for agencies interested in preparing for a potential avalanche of requests relating to the expected dramatic increase in available genetic-related information. One way to confront these issues is to provide the public the skills and resources that build their sense of efficacy when

continued

BOX 3.4.   *Continued*

confronted with these problems. In situations of high fear and worry, efficacy becomes critical to insuring constructive responses to problems (Witte, 1992). An example of a dysfunctional outcome is suicidal ideation and actual suicide in the case of Huntington's chorea (Wahlin, 2007). On the one hand, reactions to positive test results can cause feelings of extreme dismay or suicidal tendencies (Marteau & Croyle, 1998), and on the other, negative test results may have the unintended effect of people acting in unhealthy ways due to false reassurance or misinterpretation of results (Armstrong et al., 2002).

The literature suggests potentially high levels of interest in obtaining personal genetic information. However, it also suggests that conventional approaches to providing genetic counseling may not greatly diminish perceptions of risk, even among those at low risk (Croyle & Lerman, 1999). It also suggests that new ways must be found to deliver this information in an accessible and culturally sensitive way to underserved populations (Durfy et al., 1999; Lerman et al., 1999; Ludman et al., 1999). This, coupled with the shortage of cancer genetic counselors (Rothstein, 1997), the international controversy over whether general practitioners can assume this role (Bottorff et al., 1998), and emerging legal issues relating to genetics (Stopfer, 2000), suggests that any significant increase in the public's interest and requests will need to be borne by frontline caregivers.

Another set of empirical findings that compels us to advance theory relates to the paradoxical decline in the desire for information as one's proximity to a problem increases. It has been suggested that one of the shibboleth's of the communication discipline needs to be rethought: that there is not a universal desire for uncertainty reduction but rather a need for individuals to manage their uncertainty (Babrow, 2001). This is coupled with an interest in the whole area of information avoidance (Brashers, Goldsmith & Hsieh, 2002; D. O. Case et al., 2005). The essential point is that people will arrange their information environment in a manner that is consonant with their personal predispositions (J. D. Johnson, 1997). Genetic information can be very disquieting, and there may be low efficacy, since there is little one can do to ameliorate its consequences: as a result individuals often avoid information (e.g., the results of a genetic test) as their proximity to a disease increases (J. D. Johnson, Andrews & Allard, 2001).

Increasingly, individualized choices related to genetic information seeking are going to have profound implications for people's morbidity and mortality. These private choices are also going to have societal implications in the increasingly likely world of "privatized eugenics." The infrastructure to support these individual decisions is just now developing, supported by a ubiquitous Internet that increases the cacophony of voices related to any genetic issues (D. Case et al., 2004). Existing institutional resources (e.g., overburdened genetic counselors, busy family practitioners) are unlikely to be able to respond to projected demand attendant to the "mainstreaming of genetics into the practice of medicine" (F. S. Collins & McKusick, 2001). This makes it more likely that new sources will be developed, some of which we can only roughly anticipate. Finally, as Condit (1999) has clearly identified, societies have critical interests in how genetic issues are approached. So, individual choices (e.g., cloning, use of stem-cell technology) will increasingly be constrained by policy, regulatory, and governmental decision making, driven by influence attempts of an increasing range of advocacy groups. While, somewhat uniquely, the human genome project from its outset has been concerned with the ethical, legal, and social implications of this tremendous set of scientific advances (F. S. Collins et al., 2003), it is fair to say that institutional responses have lagged, in part because of the continued funding crisis in our health care system. This leads to a paradox: the more personalized the medicine, the less likely business is to be interested because there is not a scale large enough to return a profit.

FURTHER READINGS

Altman, I., & Taylor, D. A. (1973). *Social penetration: The development of interpersonal relationships.* New York: Holt, Rinehart and Winston.

Very influential work on the development of intimacy in interpersonal relationships.

Bochner, A. P. (1982). On the efficacy of openness in close relationships. In M. Burgoon (Ed.), *Communication yearbook 5* (pp. 109–144). New Brunswick, NJ: Transaction Books.

Bochner and Parks (see below), in adjacent articles in *Communication Yearbook 5*, wrote very detailed arguments against the dominant paradigm of self-disclosure in relationships, detailing the potential costs that disclosure could have. Bochner's chapter also details different dimensions of disclosure.

Epstein, R. M., & Street, R. L., Jr. (2007). *Patient-centered communication in cancer care: Promoting healing and reducing suffering.* (NIH Publication No. 07-6225). Bethesda, MD: National Institutes of Health.

Comprehensive treatment of the state-of-the-art in physician-patient interactions sponsored by the National Cancer Institute.

Marwell, G., & Schmitt, D. R. (1967). Dimensions of compliance gaining behavior: An empirical analysis. *Sociometry, 30,* 350–364.

This research inspired a very influential group of scholars with ties to Michigan State University to focus on strategies associated with intentional approaches to interpersonal influence.

Parks, M. R. (1982). Ideology in interpersonal communication: Off the couch and into the world. In M. Burgoon (Ed.), *Communication yearbook 5* (pp. 79–107). New Brunswick, NJ: Transaction Books.

Bochner (see above) and Parks, at roughly the same time, wrote very detailed arguments against the dominant paradigm of self-disclosure in relationships, detailing the potential costs that disclosure could have. Parks was especially interested in the ways values affect scientific work.

Petronio, S. (2002). *Boundaries of privacy: Dialectics of disclosure.* Albany: State University of New York Press.

A systematic bringing together of Petronio's decades-long research program focused on the boundaries of privacy. Increasingly her work is being extended to applied settings, especially those focused on health concerns.

• *4* •

Interprofessional Teams

$\mathcal{G}$roups take many forms in health care settings: grand rounds, research groups, communities of practice, nominal care groups, ad hoc groups, interdisciplinary teams, and on and on. They also serve a range of critical functions: sense making, creating knowledge, sharing it, distributing it, and collaborating. Given the complexity of our health care system, increasingly the operation of interdisciplinary teams is critical to health care outcomes, and this will be the focus of this chapter.

The impact of internal organizational grouping has always been of central interest to organizational behavior, dating back at least to the Hawthorne studies, which clearly demonstrated that informal groups had profound effects on organizational performance (Kilduff & Tsai, 2003; Scott, 2000). In the 1950s and 1960s there was a considerable body of work focused on the issue of how small group communication structures impacted performance and member satisfaction (Shaw, 1971). After a long fallow period, work on group networks within organizations has focused on the balance between internal and external information ties, dosages of different sorts, needed to achieve optimal work performance (Katz et al., 2004). While traditionally communication has been recognized as the functional means by which groups accomplish goals, increasingly groups are seen as constituted by the communication their members have with each other, which may be even more critical to the operation of interprofessional teams.

Although a variety of metaphors (e.g., pawns, puppets, hunting packs) have been applied to the study of group communication (J. T. Wood & Phillips, 1980), in an interesting convention paper Michael Holmes (1994) argued, following Scott Poole, that one of the reasons group communication research was becoming moribund was that it lacked compelling metaphors. He argued that the most compelling one in the 1990s was the "group as

35

thinker." This in part relates to the focus on decision making and creative problem solving that we will touch on in this chapter. Less attention was paid to the "group as actor" metaphor, which may be much more pertinent to the operation of interprofessional health teams. This metaphor focuses us on such issues as intragroup specialization, coordination, integration toward common goals, task completion, leadership, accountability, and so on. This view also draws attention to the centrality of communication in accomplishing work. In a way, a focus on teams for group research is itself a metaphor.

TEAMWORK

> Teams have a well-defined focus and a sense of purpose and unity that members of other groups do not share (Poole & Real, 2003, p. 370).

Teams have been important elements of health care delivery for over 100 years, with accelerating usage over the last couple decades as technology has continued to rapidly develop and medical care has grown more complex (Poole & Real, 2003). A number of different labels have been applied to the interdisciplinary teams we will focus on. For example, transdisciplinary teams engage in teaching and learning across disciplinary boundaries, promoting information sharing and collaboration resulting from a high degree of trust (Poole & Real, 2003). These different labels often point to the potential benefits of interdisciplinary teams, including the many different types of expertise and points of view that are brought to the table, greater access to a wider range of resources outside the team, shared risks and outcomes, greater commitment to achievement of overall goals, and greater learning and potential growth among team members.

In spite of their pervasiveness there are still numerous problems with the operation of teams in medical care settings: professional silos, poor communication, rigid roles, generally disappointing performance (Poole & Real, 2003), incompatible communication styles, negative team norms, power differentials, and role conflict (Quinlan, 2009). (See box 4.1 on coordinating care). Ironically, in part because of the difficulties inherent in sharing tacit knowledge dialogically across professional boundaries, teams may ultimately be less efficient in delivering medical care (Quinlan, 2009). Fundamentally, the very essence of a profession is implicated in its control of knowledge and dominating outsiders who would undermine this control (Abbott, 1988). The relationships between diverse professional groupings, who jealously guard their domains, is an increasingly critical problem, particularly in health care settings (Clarke & Everest, 2006; D'Amour et al., 2005). The work of interprofessional teams directly confronts this guiding principle of professional life. Just because one is assigned

BOX 4.1.   COORDINATING PATIENT CARE

Figure 4.1 portrays the communication network surrounding a patient with circles representing individuals and lines indicating their communication relationships. Often interprofessional teams are constituted around patients, so this diagram is instructive of the dynamics of typical problems they confront. It also, sadly, is a considerable oversimplification of the complex relationships confronting anyone who experiences a serious and/or chronic illness. All too often it is the patient who is left to coordinate his or her own care, so we will take this as the starting point for our discussion in this box.

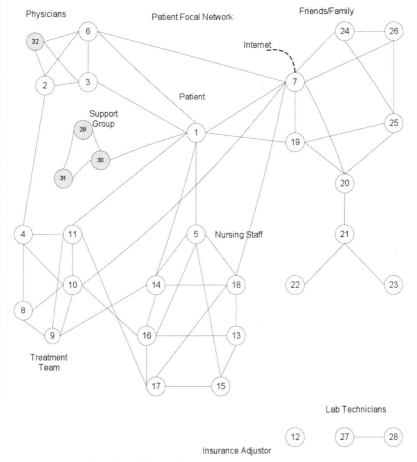

Figure 4.1.   Patient Focal Network

continued

BOX 4.1.   *Continued*

Patients in a network configured like the one in figure 4.1 can quickly become overwhelmed with the stress and information-processing demands confronting them. Not only do they have to cope with their own personal reactions to illness and, perhaps, diminished energy and cognitive abilities, but they essentially are the gatekeepers and relayers of information among the various groups they are in contact with.

Recognizing this, hospitals and other medical institutions are developing various navigator roles that assist the patient in these endeavors, but they often do not capture the full complexity of this network. So they often omit the role of patient support groups, especially online ones like PatientsLikeMe that provide considerable social support as well as medical information. They also tend not to systematically incorporate family members. Network members 7 and 19 are positioned in such a way that they can buffer the patient from some of the demands of their family members and friends.

Typically, then, interprofessional teams incorporate the physicians, treatment team, nursing staff, and perhaps other professionals like the insurance adjustor and lab technicians identified in the figure. In figure 4.1 the patient by default is the liaison that ties all of these groups together. The promise of interprofessional teams is that they will relieve patients of this coordinating role as well as insure more direct communication with each other so everyone treating the patient is on the same page.

to a work group does not mean that the group will function as a team (Poole & Real, 2003), which leads us to the obstacles to interdisciplinarity.

Obstacles to Interdisciplinarity

"Structural secrecy" refers to the way division of labor, hierarchy and specialization segregate knowledge. . . . Structural secrecy implies that (a) information and knowledge will always be partial and incomplete, (b) the potential for things to go wrong increases when tasks or information cross internal boundaries, and (c) segregated knowledge minimizes the ability to detect and stave off activities that deviate from normative standards and expectations (Vaughan, 1999, p. 277).

How people categorize their social world into affiliative groups is critical to how they go about searching for information in a directed fashion, since the first step will often embed certain assumptions about the types of people likely to have certain kinds of knowledge (Watts, 2003). Highly dense, relatively isolated cliques can be expected to have high levels of tacit knowledge, while overlapping is critical to the sharing of knowledge and development of common perspectives throughout an entire organization. The overlap of clique membership (Katz et al., 2004; Kilduff & Tsai, 2003) and the relative continuity of relationships in often fractured social systems, such as virtual organizations, often make a clear identification of groupings difficult.

One of the fundamental paradoxes of organizational life is that the greater the effort to develop deep, tacit, specialized knowledge, which often results from high connectiveness and density, the less likely it is that innovations will spread. Intergroup collaboration is often dependent on finding common frameworks in which people can interact. While we are steadily increasing our knowledge of specific subareas, we are also raising the dilemma of decreasing the possibility of any one person knowing enough about each of the parts to integrate the whole (Thayer, 1988). Specialization also limits the possibility of improvements along a technological trajectory (e.g., disruptive innovations), leads to rigidity, and often experiences diminishing returns (Katila & Ahuja, 2002). There is a finite limit to the number of new ideas that can be produced from the same elements of a knowledge set (Katila & Ahuja, 2002). Accordingly, the operation of interprofessional teams may facilitate creativity and the transfer of new knowledge across professional groups, thus facilitating the dissemination of innovations associated with clinical and translational science, which we will discuss in much more detail in chapter 7.

However, there has been considerable debate over whether teams composed of different professionals can truly achieve the level of collaboration that modern health care and clinical and translational science would seem to require. This is reflected in the distinctions between multidisciplinary, interdisciplinary, and transdisciplinary approaches to health communication (Parrott & Kreuter, 2011). Multidisciplinary approaches reflect work of a group that is done independently by group members operating from their own professional framework. Interdisciplinary work involves more direct collaboration and joint efforts moving to the more truly team-like work of transdisciplinary approaches. These efforts are more truly integrative and can reflect unique, innovative syntheses of various professional approaches. However, these approaches often involve considerable start-up costs in developing common grounds (Stokols, 2006) based on shared understandings and common histories that group members have constituted through their communication activities.

Bridging Professional Worlds

Fundamentally a focus on interprofessional teams is also a story about how different social worlds instantiated in different social groupings are bridged. Ron Burt's (1992, 2000, 2007) concept of structural holes can be fruitfully applied to this problem since it starts with relatively isolated groupings that might reflect different specialties. Structural holes are gaps or separations in communication network relationships and are framed as "disconnections or nonequivalencies between players in an arena" (Burt, 1992, pp. 1–2). Structural holes normally exist in a functioning network since network members do not share equal access to information or resources (Burt, 1992).

These discontinuities in a social structure create opportunities for interdisciplinarity, but they require individuals with unique skills to bridge them. For example, if two formal divisions that need to interact in a hospital (e.g., surgical units and nursing) do not have formal integration links, then the individuals in these units who establish informal bridge or liaison linkages have an advantage over their fellows in providing quality care to patients. Individuals can turn such relationships into "social capital," which gives them strategic advantage. A special case of brokerage comes when a person brokers relationships between asymmetrical groups, which are often found in the interrelationships between various medical professionals.

Essentials of Teamwork

It has been estimated that over 30% of operating teams' communication could be characterized as a failure in some way, often because of failures to match the amount of communication to the task at hand (Firth-Cozens, 2004), and a third of these failures jeopardized patient safety by increasing cognitive load, interrupting routine, and increasing tensions in operating rooms (Lingard et al., 2004). Health care teams take on some of the characteristics of negotiated temporary systems with frequent changes in group composition and communication linkages, less hierarchical emergent group structures, and group relationships that are embedded in a broader external system (Walker & Stohl, 2012). These systems may start bumping into the upper limits of the abilities of individuals and the groups they are embedded in to effectively process information (Walker & Stohl, 2012).

Effective health care teams are characterized by external support; appropriate member attributes (e.g., knowledge and skills); effective interpersonal relationships; organizational attributes (e.g., leadership, defined roles, goals, and so on); attention to process, particularly its communication elements (Hirokawa, DeGooyer, & Valde, 2003); interdependence; flexibility; collective ownership of goals; a history of collaboration; and reflection on process (Bronstein, 2003; Stokols, 2006). Matching the complexity of the team's membership to the complexity of the task at hand is often the key to successful outcomes, with greater adaptability, decentralization, and autonomy critical for more complex tasks (Poole & Real, 2003). These numerous conditions necessary for team success point to the difficulty of attaining the vision of interprofessional teams (Stokols, 2006). (See box 4.2.) Work groups, in general, in organizations have been estimated to be less than 20% effective in contributing to an organization's goals (Myers, Shimotsu, & Claus, 2013).

One important characteristic of effective health care teams is that doctors allow themselves to become a partner rather than a dictator (Edmondson, Bohmer, & Pisano, 2001), thereby minimizing status and power differentials within a team and promoting reciprocal respect of the status of the professions involved (Bronstein, 2003). Strategies for changing physicians' behavior and performance that embed them within teams have shown some promise in improving health care outcomes (Grol, 2002). Leaderless teams, such as communities of practice (CoP), detailed in box 4.3, have been pointed to as an exemplar that could be followed.

BOX 4.2. FACTORS PROMOTING TEAM EFFECTIVENESS

There are a number of factors that contribute to the effectiveness of teams, with perhaps a modification of Tolstoy's famous observation about families in order. All effective teams may be similarly configured, but there is a multiplicity of patterns that can result in ineffective teams. One essential overall principle that must be in place for overall team effectiveness is that the team must match in some way the task at hand. Unfortunately teams often represent overdoses, which leads to frustration and low morale.

In terms of exogenous, or input, variables, teams should be of appropriate size with a mix of specialists needed to perform the task at hand. They need to have the support of the institutions within which they are embedded and the appropriate resources needed for accomplishing their task. They must have sufficient time to devote to the accomplishment of their goal.

Internal group processes must also be aligned with appropriate levels of cohesion; there must be a clear understanding of group structure and how internal decisions within the group will be reached; a high degree of respect and trust should be present; destructive practices such as social loafing and groupthink should be minimized; appropriate conflict resolution strategies should be followed; there should be some common ground essential for effective communication; there should be clear goals and a rational for teams' existence; routines and practices should reinforce group goals; progress and outcomes measures should be in place to insure accountability; the group should reflect on practice; and, finally, equitable member contributions and participation should be insured. This rather long list of things necessary for success again points to the difficulty of developing truly effective interprofessional teams.

BOX 4.3.   COMMUNITIES OF PRACTICE

Within a CoP, people collaborate directly; teach each other; and share experiences and knowledge in ways that foster innovation (Smith & McKeen, 2003, p. 395).

The operation of communities of practice (CoPs) has been increasingly central to our understanding of how diverse groups of professionals come together to improve practice and implement innovations (Leonard, 2006; Wenger, McDermott & Snyder, 2002).

CoPs often discourage hierarchical relationships within their community, and the community generates its own goals (E. L. Lesser & Storck, 2004). CoPs are formed by groups of people who share tacit knowledge and/or learn through experimentation focusing on central organizational processes or problems (Brown & Duguid, 2002; E. Lesser & Prusak, 2004; Tidd, 2000). CoPs form around communities of people who have areas of common interest (e.g., practices) within a domain and exchange information that result in improvements in the whole (Fontaine, 2004; Huysman & van Baalen, 2002; E. L. Lesser & Storck, 2004; Wenger, McDermott & Snyder, 2002).

These communities are particularly important for geographically dispersed, virtual organizations (Scarbrough & Swan, 2002). Increasingly attention has turned to ever more complex forms of communities, such as those involved in developing open source software. In examining the case of Linux, Lee and Cole (2003) noted the importance of critique in these communities for error identification, correction, and rejection that was critical to the evolution of knowledge.

INTERDEPENDENCE

Question conventional wisdom that teamwork is inherently good and that the more there is of it the better off the team will be (Crawford & Lepine, 2013, p. 33).

Since it is impossible to keep track of developments in a wide variety of professional arenas, team members depend on each other to bring their expertise related to these developments to the table (Reddy & Spence, 2008). Interdependence, along with flexibility, collective ownership of goals, and reflection on process, has been seen to play a key role in interprofessional collaboration for social workers (Bronstein, 2003). It is a necessary consequence of the division of labor in an organization (Victor & Blackburn, 1987). The "group as actor" metaphor focuses us on the coordinated actions of interdependent actors (Holmes, 1994).

J. D. Thompson's (1967) classification of differing types of interdependencies associated with technology has implicit linkages to the dosage metaphor. Thompson (1967) sees structure as facilitating coordinated action among interdependent elements of the organization. Each of the following types of interdependence he identified is generally characteristic of particular groups, although they can also contain preceding types. A fundamental insight of contingency approaches is that groups must match their level of interdependence to the task at hand (Lawrence & Lorsch, 1967; Woodward, 1965). Interdependencies are reflected in a variety of coordination mechanisms (e.g., routines, meetings, schedules, direct hierarchical contact) in which communication is centrally implicated (Okhuysen & Bechky, 2009), with true collaboration, as we have seen, often entailing considerable costs. In turn, the limits of coordination may limit the degree of specialization in organizations (Becker & Murphy, 1992). The failure to match network relationships (e.g., strong ties with reciprocal interdependence) to particular types of interdependence is likely to result in coordination failures (Gargiulo & Benassi, 2000).

In pooled interdependence each part of a system renders a discrete contribution and is supported by the whole (e.g., a track team). Pooled interdependence, which is coordinated by standardization, also implies low levels of communication (e.g., medical supply people who fill requests by standardized orders).

When one unit of the organization must act before another can, you have sequential interdependence (e.g., an assembly line) with direct analogs to the dosage element of sequencing. Coordination by plan characterizes sequential interdependence. It requires more communication, particularly with adjacent individuals and to control adherence to the plan, but it implies a one-way flow of communication messages. Typically sequential interdependence (e.g., characteristic of some surgical units where you have pre-op, the operation itself, and then recovery) requires that workers be bound to work stations and/or equipment for much of the day. In assembly-line operation this is not a block to all interactions but rather limits it to those others with overlapping information fields. Thus, Form (1972) found a high frequency of interaction among proximate others in an assembly-line operation, but the nature of the technology resulted in short, relatively shallow interactions.

Reciprocal interdependence, often reflected in the operation of true teams, is found when the outputs of each element of the system become inputs for others. Reciprocal interdependence units (e.g., surgical trauma teams), should be much more fluid in their operations with less formally directed coordination links and less routine, directed tasks. The coordination by mutual adjustment necessary for reciprocal interdependence requires high degrees of feedback and thus implies a two-way flow of messages. "There is a maximum point at which the benefits of increased coordination become overwhelmed by the costs of communication" (Crawford & Lepine, 2013, p. 37). This has led to a focus on implicit coordination where teams dynamically adjust their behavior without directly communicating with each other. This sort of minimalist approach to communication is often required in decision making and self-organizing action teams (Rico et al., 2008).

As we proceed along the different types of interdependence and associated coordination modes, the costs of communication and the burdens of decision making increase (J. D. Thompson, 1967). Each of the types of interdependence also imply different levels of coordination costs for the parties (Gulati, 2007). Under norms of rationality and efficiency, organizations will try to minimize the need for more complicated modes of coordination and interdependence, such as those found in transdisciplinary teams, in the process reducing the need for repeated doses of communication but perhaps leading to reduced efficacy over time.

STRESS AND BURNOUT

> Excessive teamwork imposes communication burdens that may distract members from accomplishing tasks (Crawford & Lepine, 2013, p. 44).

Of course, pressures to move to teamwork and to higher levels of interdependence can increase the tensions and conflicts already being experienced by health care workers. Stress and burnout are all too common among them since they often face emotional exhaustion from the very nature of their work. They also are associated with workload, and thus to dosage issues (Miller, Zook, & Ellis, 1989) and associated with a high desire to leave one's job and a lack of emotional responsiveness to clients (J. Snyder, 2009). One key communication strategy often suggested for coping with these problems is to activate someone's surrounding social network to provide needed support. It is seen as being "inextricably woven into communication behavior" (Albrecht & Adelman, 1987c, p. 14).

"Social support refers to verbal and nonverbal communication between recipients and providers that reduces uncertainty about the situation, the self, the other, or the relationship, and functions to enhance a perception of personal control in one's life experience" (Albrecht & Adelman, 1987a, p. 19).

Generally two crucial dimensions of support are isolated, informational and emotional, with informational support associated with a feeling of mastery and control over one's environment (Freimuth, 1987) and emotional support crucial to feelings of personal coping, enhanced self-esteem, and needs for affiliation (Albrecht & Adelman, 1987b) and more likely to be important in coping with burnout associated with emotional contagion (Ray & Apker, 2011). The level of support has been associated with such critical outcomes as stress, absenteeism, burnout, turnover, productivity, and worker morale (Ray, 1987).

While individuals to whom an individual is strongly tied may be more readily accessible and more willing to be of assistance (Granovetter, 1982), the social support literature has often focused on weak ties as a major form of support. This again focuses us on matching issues and assuring that the proper level of dosage is given for particular problems people may be confronting. Weak ties provide critical informational support because they transcend the limitations of our strong ties and because our strong ties can be disrupted or unavailable (Adelman, Parks, & Albrecht, 1987). Weak ties may be useful for discussing things you do not want to reveal to your close work associates, providing a place for an individual to experiment, extending access to information, promoting social comparison, and fostering a sense of community (Adelman, Parks, & Albrecht, 1987).

Networks are often viewed as the infrastructure of social support (Albrecht & Adelman, 1987b). For example, Albrecht, Irey, & Mundy (1982) found that workers who spent much of their time outside the organization needed to be highly integrated into their organizations. The literature on the relationship between integratedness (couched in network terms), support, and burnout is probably the most developed in this area. However, the results of the studies that have been done are somewhat mixed (Ray, 1987), providing some interesting insights into the dysfunctional aspects of support.

Of course, people other than health professionals need supportive communication, and it often plays a critical role in medical treatment, especially in uncertainty management (Goldsmith & Albrecht, 2011). Increasingly attention has also shifted to caregivers and their needs for support. It has been suggested that caregivers would be helped by "a sufficiency in the amount or dosage of treatment" (Zarit & Femia, 2008, p. 47), with others wondering what a "therapeutic 'dose' of social or instrumental support" might be to allow a family to continue caregiving for one of its members (Given, Given, & Kozachik, 2001, p. 222).

Early studies in this area tended to argue that the more integrated networks were, the more supportive they were (Albrecht, 1982). Indeed, high-density networks tend to lead to positive social identity and the acquisition of tangible services from others with whom the individual has strong ties (Albrecht & Adelman, 1987c). However, it turns out that less dense networks of relationships may be more supportive, since they provide access to a wider range of information sources (Ray, 1987). High-density networks can also be stifling and even devastating for individuals who are rejected by their groups (Albrecht & Adelman, 1987b). They may also be stressful because their maintenance requires more energy (Ray, 1987). These assertions are supported by a study conducted by Kirmeyer and Lin (1987), which found a negative relationship between communication with peers and social support. In terms of larger system consequences, highly integrated networks run the risk of dysfunctional social contagion effects, since, for example, stressed individuals may increase the stress of others (decreasing the support they in turn can give), putting the whole system at risk (Albrecht & Adelman, 1987c).

In summary, individuals in low-density, heterogeneous networks, partitioned into discrete subfunctions, often fare better in terms of social support. In particular, ties to others outside the immediate work unit are much more likely to reduce burnout and stress (Albrecht, 1982; Ray, 1987), which may be a side benefit of interprofessional teams. These networks facilitate coping, role transition, and access to needed information (Albrecht & Adelman, 1987b). They also contribute to a greater sense of personal control on the part of individuals, since they are not dependent on any one group of individuals (Albrecht & Adelman, 1987b). Not so paradoxically then, Leiter (1988) has found that at higher levels work-related contacts may be associated with both increased feelings of personal accomplishment and increased emotional exhaustion among members of a multidisciplinary mental health team.

While the social support literature focuses on communication networks, recent attention has shifted to online support groups (Wright et al., 2011). This is a somewhat limited view of the array of supports offered by the formal structure of an organization, particularly because such organizational features as the length of tenure of employees and the extent to which a particular position permits interaction limit the role networks play in social support (Ray, 1987). Many formal organizational programs, often fostered within the perspective of human relations approaches, are specifically designed to achieve social-support-related outcomes. Employee assistance programs and mentoring programs are examples of formal organizational mechanisms designed to support the employee.

Communication networks themselves can represent convergence of network members around symbolic meanings of support (Albrecht & Adelman, 1987b). This highlights the importance of context in the development of supportive relationships, since supportive relationships may be best provided by those who share a particular context, and stable relationships are also more likely to be supportive (Ray, 1987). These networks can in effect constitute elaborate feedback processes through which individual behavior is regulated and maintained, often through concertative control mechanisms. At times, such as with drug addicts in larger societal settings, the enmeshment of individuals in these networks may not be to anyone's benefit (Albrecht & Adelman, 1987b).

Other elements of an organization and/or a profession's culture may also play a role in the development of supportive relationships. Support within organizations can exist only to the extent organizations are committed to a supportive climate symbolically and tangibly (Ray, 1987). For example, root metaphors of an organizational culture can greatly influence whether or not support is offered and what type will be given. A family metaphor is inherently a supportive one, while other metaphors, such as the machine, where an individual is viewed as an interchangeable part, are antithetical to support. Also, the normative rule structure of an organization may affect the willingness of others to give support.

FRAMEWORKS

Developing a common understanding, something that is also centrally important to communication more generally, is central to effective coordination (Okhuysen & Bechky, 2009). Often this common understanding, or ground, is based on larger frameworks in which individuals are embedded. Frameworks have been used in a variety of social sciences (e.g., L. L. Putnam & Holmer, 1992; Schon & Rein, 1994; Tversky & Kahneman, 1981), especially in work focused on discourse processes (Bateson, 1972; Goffman, 1974). They indicate a way both of viewing the world and of interpreting it in sense making (Gray, 1996).

Here we will focus on frameworks that provide a more encompassing context for interaction within interdisciplinary teams. A framework for interaction is the set of interrelated conditions that promote certain levels of shared understanding of meanings, orient interactants to the nature of the event, and establish the ultimate purpose of continuing interaction (J. D. Johnson, 1997b, 1998). A framework, then, is the ground that opens doors to social worlds of situated knowledge and governing rationalities, providing a programmed way of approaching problems often embodied in organizational routines. Frameworks serve a number of functions: they provide shared conversational resources, establish a common emotional tone, insure quicker responses (Collins, 1981), and provide a basis for temporal stability (Benson, 1975; Collins, 1981). They interact with doses to promote receptivity to some messages, while making some others more difficult to understand. Four frameworks—formal, informal, markets, and professional—are particularly important for the operation of interprofessional teams.

Formal approaches (e.g., organizational design and bureaucracy) rely heavily on explicit knowledge and well-understood code systems, but they are often incomplete and ignore social factors represented in informal communication. Both formal and informal frameworks appeal to different metaphors, mechanistic and organismic, respectively (J. D. Johnson, 1993a; Morgan, 1986). Usually formal frameworks require only a limited form of understanding, based on system rules, training, and a legalistic understanding of relationships between positions. Actors are presupposed to be governed by the requirements of the positions they occupy in an organization's formal structure.

The growth of IT and global competition has pushed the envelope of formal structures, with contemporary writers focusing on the virtual characteristics of structure and giving increasing importance to knowledge-related issues in the operation of interprofessional teams. These forces also draw our attention to other frameworks that exist in contemporary, complex health organizations. Exchange rests on individuals pursuing their rational self-interest as in markets, while culturally related normative frameworks depend on operations of larger collectivities most clearly represented in the professions.

Markets focus on exchange relationships and the paramount importance of trust in characterizing them. Trust, in turn, greatly facilitates the receptivity of any message. Obviously, an exchange relationship can rest on extremely rudimentary understandings of others, based on such fundamental issues as fair price and a belief that the other party will follow through on bargains. Relationships are seen from a utilitarian perspective, with the primary bases for continued relationships resulting from a perception of mutual gain. Markets, through the mechanisms of exchanges, operate to diffuse information rapidly to interested parties (F. von Hayek, 1991) in an overall configuration often cast as traders in a bazaar (Geertz, 1973). Markets have an inherently dynamic view of information exchanges, with individuals compelled to change their ideas as a result of the reactions of others. In this view organizations are islands of planned coordination relationships, often revealed in intragroup communication, perhaps represented by professions to which we know turn, embedded in a sea of market relationships (Powell, 1990).

In some ways health organizations have become umbrellas for various professional guilds. They come together to pursue loosely defined larger objectives (e.g., universities and the pursuit of knowledge). So, these organizations are splintered into different functional groupings and "occupational communities" that form subcultures (Amabile et al., 2001; Gregory, 1983; J.

D. Johnson, 1993; Keller, 2001). Relationships between and among professions are often governed by normative expectations (Cheney & Ashcraft, 2007).

Most work on the professions has focused on how they establish (and protect) their jurisdictions and maintain their status within broader social systems. Knowledge is seen as a key tool in these processes (Abbott, 1988; Lammers & Garcia, 2009; Macdonald, 1995), especially in regard to "special competence in esoteric bodies of knowledge linked to central needs and values of the social system" (Larson, 1977, p. xi). Knowledge is intimately related with credentialing and training and the formal (and often legal, state-enforced) differentiation of specialties in societies generally and organizations specifically (Macdonald, 1995). Once true expertise is developed, the professional may have a very difficult time translating it for the novice or generalist (Hinds & Pfeffer, 2003). Professions also develop strong norms of "purity" that impede their ability to confront new, ambiguous problems (Abbott, 1981), such as those that are often the focus of interprofessional teams.

A key element of this socialization is the development of elaborate semantic systems of tacit understandings (F. A. von Hayek, 1945) that are difficult to share. The more elaborate and refined the framework, the more effective the communication within the profession (and the more difficult outside it). An advantage of strong cultures is their enhancement of shared understandings between actors and a norm of adjustment through consultation within a system of mutual authority that governs competition (Polanyi & Prosch, 1975).

One of the basic problems with relying exclusively on what goes on within an organization is that there is a finite limit to the number of new ideas that can be produced from the same elements of a knowledge set (Katila & Ahuja, 2002). Professions play a unique role in determining where substantive change within organizations comes from. In many ways strong professions transcend particular organizations and make their boundaries more permeable. Membership in a profession provides access to a much larger, scalable tacit knowledge community outside the organization (Lammers & Garcia, 2009). These much broader tacit networks, especially those associated with professional institutions, become the primary vehicle for external learning (Lammers & Garcia, 2009; Van der Krogt, 1998).

The relationships among diverse professional groupings, which jealously guard their domains, is an increasingly critical problem, particularly in health care settings (Clark, 2006; D'Amour et al., 2005). "Professionals tend to pursue their own aspirations and to maintain their professional autonomy and jurisdiction rather than opening their practice to collaborative behavior" (Sicotte, D'Amour, & Moreault, 2002). However, balancing cooperation and

BOX 4.4.   MINGLING DECISION-MAKING METAPHORS

The existence of multiple cultures and their configuration into coalitions can be taken as a given in most organizations (Morgan, 1986). Perhaps the crucial question is whether or not there is a dominant culture or a more pluralistic arrangement of subcultures. One way in which subcultures may relate to each other at the deeper levels of culture is through the usage of metaphors, which are essential to communicating the frameworks in which they operate.

Meyer's (1984) research on the use of metaphors related to coalitions in a hospital setting is very interesting in this regard. He argues that in hospitals there are four dominant root metaphors that serve as decision-making models for different coalitions: organism (physicians), computation (administrators, government agencies), cybernetics (boards of directors), and pluralism (the interaction of major coalitions). In making decisions concerning medical equipment, it is unlikely that one of these metaphors can totally dominate. What is needed is an overlap of argument that can make symbolic sense in the context of more than one framework. Thus coalitions are built on the overlap of symbol systems as well as relationships, the "big tent" in political systems (e.g., the New Deal, the Reagan Revolution), that can provide an encompassing framework for disparate groups. So, equipment that serves long-term strategic interests, has a substantial return on investment, and benefits patients is more likely to appeal to a cross section of hospital subcultures.

competition must be achieved, most notably in sharing information that is in the interest of the collective, in spite of individual motivations to hoard (Kalman et al., 2002). Often members operating in different frames need to come together to accomplish larger, collective purposes. As we have seen, these issues are critical to the operation of interprofessional teams. Decision making, which we turn to next, often rests on the cooperative judgments of organizational members immersed in different frameworks, and it is also reflected in box 4.4, which focuses on decision making related to hospital purchases.

DECISION MAKING

The greater the group discussion, the more likely it is that information needed for effective decision making will be distributed widely and applied in problem solving. Higher levels of discussion also make it more likely members will detect errors and correct them, improving individual cognition and performance (Hirokawa, 1996). While there have been numerous models of group decision making proposed, here we will focus as an exemplar on that developed by Gouran and Hirokawa (2003), the Functional Perspective on Group Decision Making. This theory predicts when a group will make a high-quality decision. They argue that high-quality decisions result when groups rationally, in part by sticking to requisite tasks in their internal communication, address four essential functions: analyze the problem, set goals, identify alternatives, and evaluate both positive and negative consequences of these alternatives. Often cultures and/or frameworks are deeply implicated in all of these functions.

The Impact of Multiple Frameworks

Early approaches to culture tended to assume that there was one culture within an organization, or at least a dominant one, usually identified with management (Deal & Kennedy, 1982). Indeed, from this perspective culture becomes a variable management can manipulate for its own ends (Smircich & Calas, 1987). While comforting to management, this perspective vastly oversimplifies life in modern, complex organizations. In fact, some of the early classics of organizational research, such as the Hawthorne studies, involved the recognition of subcultures within organizations.

The existence of multiple cultures and their configuration into coalitions can be taken as a given in most organizations (Eisenberg, Contractor, & Monge, 1988; Morgan, 1986). These subcultures are often associated with coalitions and political processes. Communication across subgroups is often difficult and subject to distortion because of the different language schemas, goal orientations, and task differentiations that become embodied in the metaphors they select and how they apply them (see box 4.4). Perhaps the crucial question relates to whether or not there is a dominant subculture or more of a pluralistic arrangement of subcultures in organizations that would seem to be the holy grail of interprofessional teams. The emergence of one form or another may be in part dependent on the duality of concerns related to collaboration and control (Frost, 1987). The weighting on these dimensions can determine the extent of pluralism in an organization, with control associated with the emergence of dominant subcultures and collaboration associated with pluralism. However, if there is in reality, as there often is in organizations like hospitals and universities, multiple, more or less equal subcultures, this heightens our concern for interprofessional communication.

These conditions also lay the ground for conflict and negotiation. Different professional groups may have different orientations to their clients (e.g., sexual assault victims, substance abusers), which often is a source of conflict in resulting treatment choices. Linda Putnam (2010) has a different take on the classic view of negotiation as focused on the outcomes of an individual who wants to achieve strategic aims. She views negotiation as "not about winning, but about meeting the needs of both parties, through generating creative options, discovering new insights, and altering the name of the game" (p. 326). This is best achieved through processes of collective sense making, such as that found in the work of true teams, often embodied in joint storytelling and the creation of new rituals.

Conflict is an inherent feature of group life, with some suggestions that a moderate level of conflict is necessary to generate new ideas and implement adequate problem solutions (Abigail & Cahn, 2013). Civilized disagreement is important for team operations, with true teams not engaging in avoiding, smoothing, or suppressing conflict as their dominant conflict resolution strategies. Often conflict results from too much communication (Abigail & Cahn, 2013), an overdose, making explicit what was once latent.

Uncertainty Management

The number of alternatives represented by frameworks inherently increases uncertainty in organizations. While early approaches to communication research focused on uncertainty reduction (Berger, 2011), most current approaches to uncertainty in health communication recognize its inevitability and stress that management of uncertainty, rather than its elimination, is the real issue. This focus on uncertainty management grew out of recognition that diseases like AIDS or HIV presented often unresolvable problems for those afflicted (Brashers et al., 2000). It is also the case that those with serious illnesses, nearing the end of life, are confronted with multiple, often overlapping uncertainties (Hines, 2001).

Concerns for sequencing and match also may determine how much information is given and when. A physician might describe a more optimistic outcome than warranted if s/he is concerned that patients will "give up hope" if they hear the unvarnished truth (Ford, Babrow, & Stohl, 1996). Patients, in turn, may avoid listening or understanding to maintain uncertainty: not knowing may be more comfortable than knowing one has a potentially fatal cancer (Brashers, Goldsmith, & Hsieh, 2002). The patient may even deliberately increase uncertainty by seeking out contradictory information (e.g., reading about alternative diagnoses and treatments or "miracle cures").

Babrow, Kasch, & Ford (1998) note that the illness experience often increases stress. They described several different senses of uncertainty extant in the literature: mental confusion, ambiguity, equivocality, equally probable alternatives, and unpredictability. They also traced major sources of uncertainty: qualities of information (e.g., clarity, accuracy, completeness, and so on), probability beliefs, and the structure of information (e.g., order, integration). They concluded that uncertainty reduction was not the exclusive motive of patients. Sometimes patients with a higher tolerance for ambiguity may be more tolerant of "watchful waiting" approaches to concerns like prostate cancer. At other times, people forestall seeking definitive diagnoses because of their potentially devastating impacts.

Creative Problem Solving

Creativity is reflected in a group's capacity to produce new ideas. This is most frequently accomplished by arranging for diverse human memberships (Perry-Smith, 2006) that are often seen as an essential precondition for creativity (Joshi, 2006). Essentially the issue of connectiveness, or density, refers to whether or not all of the possible linkages in an aggregate are being utilized. Most recent attention on this issue has focused on density, which is determined by dividing the number of actual links in a particular network by the number possible (Scott, 2000). Matching density to group tasks has become increasingly critical.

Not only are members' direct ties important, but their indirect ties permit them to experiment and scan their environment widely for information. However, without strong internal group ties, there is difficulty transferring that knowledge—the classic search transfer problem identified by Hansen (1999). The transfer of explicit codified knowledge entails that many indirect ties (which are easier to maintain) may be more beneficial than a few intensive direct ties (Ahuja, 2000). Similarly, uniplexity, or a narrow focus, facilitates information sharing by making it more likely a common perspective will develop (Mohrman, Tenkasi, & Mohrman, 2003). While these relatively dense ties with redundant others can inhibit creativity, they also build trust and cooperation, which aids tacit transfer of knowledge and influence attempts related to innovation implementation. Highly redundant linkages, a form of overdose, impair creativity, in part, because clique members have the same knowledge base, which results in similar worldviews. Increased communication, in part because it results in the development of common perspectives, and tenure, which, in addition to resulting in common perspectives, increases the likelihood of centralization and subgroup formation, have been found to decrease creativity in teams (Kratzer, Leenders, & van Engelen, 2004) and may be a rather natural process in large organizations, with the first increments of constraint more deleterious to creativity than any subsequent ones (Burt, 2005).

Generally it has been argued that diversity in perspective is a necessary precondition for creativity (Albrecht & Hall, 1989; Leonard, 2006). Diversity is a multifaceted construct, including professional training (Drazin, Glynn, &

Kazanjian, 1999), tenure, demographics, and function, which have all been related to creativity (Agrell & Gustafson, 1996). Thus, group size has been positively related to creativity, in part because it increases the potential diversity of stimuli an individual is exposed to (Agrell & Gustafson, 1996). This has led to a central focus on diversity as an essential ingredient for creativity, which can lead to creative abrasion when different perspectives are directly confronted in discourse, which can inevitably lead to conflicts that managers must anticipate (Leonard, 2006), since the very factors that can lead to creative outcomes in groups can also produce personal conflict, ineffective communication, and negative emotional reactions (Levine & Moreland, 2004).

The most common source of new product ideas is users and clients (Leonard, 2006), a form of weak tie not subject to formal influence. We will discuss in chapter 5 the dynamics in an underlying function of government information programs, where patients are given information in the hope that they will diffuse it to practitioners. Unfortunately, until the recent trends in citizen science and the broader consumer movement, the medical community has been slow to respond to this sort of influence.

Increasingly it is being recognized that there may be an underlying nonlinear, inverted, U-shaped element to these processes, with some contact (often through small world processes) necessary for stimulation, but with too much contact resulting in conformity pressures (Uzzi & Spiro, 2005). Or, stated in a different way, cohesive dense groups often become rigid, while expanding the scope of the search introduces the new, but also may introduce unreliability in organizational outputs (Katila & Ahuja, 2002). Unfortunately innovation in medical settings is often a top-down process dependent on the development of a firm evidence base, which may indeed, in the end, reduce the potential benefits of putting interprofessional teams together.

Bandwidth, Echo, and Cohesive Groups

Socially connected members of heterogeneous groups may also be more likely to self-censor their contributions than are socially isolated members, with surprisingly low proportions of good ideas being followed through on by managers who have them (Burt, 2004, 2005). (See box 4.5.) Some have argued that the first stage of decision making really rests on the frame, or knowledge base, that an individual has developed because of his or her preexisting information fields and positioning within communication structures (Carley, 1986). The communication structure an individual is embedded in is a critical part of the decision-making process, influencing the volume of information and the diversity of information sources. So we in effect are doubly vexed; the support structures we rely on for determining alternatives may have already formed the alternatives we are likely to identify.

BOX 4.5.   SPIRAL OF SILENCE

Another interesting line of research that impinges on dosage issues relates to the spiral of silence. The German social scientist Elizabeth Noelle-Neumann's (1974) work on elections noted that there is often a disparity between the distribution of public opinion and what received public voice. Interestingly, we appear to have a feel for the distributions of public opinion around us, with the question "Who do you think will win the election?" more predictive than asking individual respondents what their own position is. It appears that those who think their opinions are popular are more willing to express themselves, while those who think their opinions are unpopular will remain silent in public discussions, in part because they fear being further isolated. As time goes on this results in the spiral that makes it appear there is a more one-sided position on public issues, that there is more consensus than actually exists.

Maintaining dialog in the presence of disagreement, especially strongly held partisan beliefs, is a key element of political processes and has thus received systematic treatment in political science, with many common elements to those we discuss here (Huckfeldt, Johnson & Sprague, 2004). Processes of self-censorship, especially when one does not hold strong views, are often coupled with false consensus effects, the projection onto others of similar perspectives to one's own, that further impede convergence to commonly held underlying attitudes (Huckfeldt, Johnson & Sprague 2004). Because of the pressures to uniformity resulting from these processes, often peripheral members of organizational networks have the most creative (or, at the very least, different) perspectives (Perry-Smith & Shalley, 2003), especially when this is coupled with ties outside a social system (Perry-Smith, 2006).

As we have seen repeatedly, membership in cohesive groups results in limiting the range of considered alternatives through conformity pressures and, somewhat relatedly, the development of trusting relationships and exposure to a truly diverse range of alternatives. Group members do not share information that does not support perceived group opinions: the position of a plurality of other group members, their preferences, or the information already in the possession of other group members (Stasser & Titus, 1985).

Mind guarding acts to severely limit communication after a decision is reached: indeed, often organizational decision makers will ignore the information they have available (Feldman & March, 1981). Unfortunately, the more uncertain the information, the more subject it is to favorable distortions by those reporting it (Downs, 1967), and when information is vitally required, there is a tendency to treat it as more reliable than it actually is (Adams, 1980). Especially under conditions of threat, organizations may restrict their information seeking and fail to react to changing environmental conditions (Staw, Sandelands, & Dutton, 1981). Organizations in these circumstances rely on existing behaviors, narrow their information fields, and reduce the number of information channels consulted. In other words, they reduce dosages that may lead them to change. This, in part, explains the slow translation of evidence-based medicine into practice, which we will discuss in some detail later in chapter 6.

In terms of echo, the social system that decision makers are a part of acts to reinforce existing approaches rather than to suggest true alternatives. Decision makers are more likely to use networks to learn how to make legitimate decisions than to improve the information they use to make decisions. This creates imitative pressures that are especially likely to apply to those of lower status (March, 1994), something of great concern to the likely performance of interprofessional groups dominated by physicians. Decision makers often ask for more information (it is, after all, a part of the decision-making ritual), even when they have sufficient information on hand to make a decision (Feldman & March, 1981). They know that very seldom will they be criticized for gathering additional information, but they might be blamed for failing to gather a critical piece of information (Feldman & March, 1981), which may be reflected in the all-to-common phenomenon of unnecessary medical tests.

Information is often gathered to justify a decision already made, instead of being used to make an optimal decision (Staw, Sandelands, & Dutton, 1981). Research has repeatedly demonstrated that decision making is an irrational process. Ironically, because of forces related to bandwidth and echo (Burt, 2005), perhaps the ultimate support for the "rightness" of a decision must come from outside one's cohesive network of strong ties (Cross, Rice, & Parker, 2001).

SUMMARY AND COMMENTARY

Table 4.1 compares the elements of dosage to the various processes we have discussed in this chapter. The first two columns compare two types of collectivities, groups and teams, and suggest that the primary difference between the two is that a team represents a more intense dosage among the various elements. The other thing that is noteworthy about this table is the relative sophistication of theorizing in this area, with many contingent (it depends) statements according to the type of task confronting a group.

This is particularly true for the interdependence between group members needed to perform a task, with levels and patterns of communication

Table 4.1. Comparing Team Approaches and the Dosage Metaphor

			Approaches			
Dosage Elements	*Groups*	*Teams*	*Support*	*Interdependence*	*Frameworks*	*Decision Making*
Amount	Moderate	High	Match	Contingent	Varies	Related to uncertainty
Frequency	Moderate	High	Match	Contingent	Varies	Related to uncertainty
Sequencing	Limited	Reciprocity	Ordering	Contingent	Varies	Phases
Delivery systems	Various	Various	Social networks	Contingent	Varies	Various
Interactions	Context	Culture	Job demands	Task	Multiplexity	Uncertainty
Contraindications	Improper match	Dominant hierarchy	Contagion effects	Improper match	Dominant frame	Limited alternatives
Dysfunctions	Not a true group	Professional silos	Turnover	Overdose	Lack of common ground	Groupthink

dictated by the type of interdependence required. So it is a bad match for an interprofessional team confronted with a pooled task to encourage high levels of coordination, a clear case of overdosage, with related dysfunctions of lower morale and wasted resources.

Somewhat similarly, frameworks perspectives depend on which one is present for various actors. So actors embedded in a formal framework dependent on explicit knowledge may have relatively low levels of amount and frequency, a top-down sequencing, and a tendency toward written delivery systems, while actors embedded in markets may vary their communication levels by demand, be more reciprocal in sequencing, and rely more on truly interactive delivery systems, such as those found on a trading room floor. As we saw in the mingling decision-making metaphors box (box 4.4), health care decisions often interact with the multiplexity of frameworks present, may be contraindicated when one framework dominates, and may be dysfunctional when no common ground can be uncovered, in part because of a lack of understanding of the various frameworks that may be operative.

For support amount and frequency often rest on the proper match, with too much often leading to burnout and too little not coping with the underlying stresses individuals might feel. At times it may be necessary to sequence proper types of support first, dealing with pressing emotional concerns before following up with information needed to implement solutions. Social networks have been cast as the vehicle of supportive relationships. Health professionals often have heavy emotional burdens associated with their work, which interacts with dosage concerns. At times too much support may actually have dysfunctional consequences by contributing to contagion impacts, which may indicate situations in which support from within one's immediate networks may be contraindicated.

Finally, many consider that the ultimate purpose of interprofessional teams is to make decisions. The amount and frequency of communication necessary to do this ultimately is related to the level of uncertainty involved, a major interacting factor. As we saw in our discussion of the Functional Perspective on Group Decision Making, often there are various functions that need to be performed, which may imply some logical sequencing to group decision making. In highly complex decision-making situations, more interactive delivery systems may be preferred. A limited range of alternatives, lack of evidence, and group processes (e.g., groupthink) that impede decision making represent contraindications and dysfunctions respectively.

FURTHER READINGS

Bronstein, L. R. (2003). A model for interdisciplinary collaboration. *Social Work, 48* (3), 297–306.

Systematic discussion of components of interdisciplinary collaboration and four factors that influence it from the perspective of a social worker.

Gouran, D. S., & Hirokawa, R. Y. (2003). Effective decision making and problem solving in groups: A functional perspective. In R. Y. Hirokawa, R. S. Cathcart, L. A. Samovar & L. D. Henman (Eds.), *Small group communication: Theory and practice* (pp. 27–38). New York: Oxford University Press.

Gouran and Hirokawa argue that high-quality decisions result when groups rationally, in part by sticking to requisite tasks in their internal communication, address four essential functions: problem analysis, goal setting, identification of alternatives, and evaluation of both positive and negative consequences of these alternatives. This chapter provides a useful précis of their research program.

Katzenbach, J. R., & Smith, D. K. (1993). *The wisdom of teams: Creating the high-performance organization.* New York: HarperCollins.

The operation of teams in organizations has been the subject of numerous popular treatments. This book is a classic in this genre.

Malone, T. W., & Crowston, K. (1994). The interdisciplinary study of coordination. *ACM Computing Surveys, 26*, 87–119.

Comprehensive review of coordination issues relating to interdependence from a variety of disciplinary perspectives. Develops a framework of studying coordination and examines the increasing importance of technology in coordination work.

Perry-Smith, J. E. (2006). Social yet creative: The role of social relationships in facilitating individual creativity. *Academy of Management Journal, 49*, 85–101.

A systematic examination of the dynamic impacts of individual's social positioning on their creativity. Develops the now familiar arguments that individuals working in diverse contexts are more likely to be exposed to different and unusual ideas and that strong ties to redundant others can often result in stifling conformity.

· 5 ·

Mass Media

𝒜 variety of metaphors have been used to understand mass media: windows, interpreters, platforms, filters, mirrors, vessels (Littlejohn & Foss, 2011), cultural erosion (Varan, 1998), and the marketplace of ideas (Napoli, 1999). Historically our mass media have been institutionally based and, in broad sweep, centrally concerned with the preservation of our culture. As a result mass media theory has often focused on issues of exposure and resulting effects. The media encompass a wide array of separate channels, each with their unique properties, with at least suggestive evidence that individuals use major media differently because they find them differentially useful. The print media, such as newspapers and magazines, are more appropriate for detailed, lengthy, and technical material, while brief, simple, timely ideas are more effectively communicated via broadcast channels (Atkin, 1981; Hanneman, 1973). Television's greater intrusiveness compels exposure, but readers of newspapers[1] and magazines can readily ignore messages they encounter (Atkin, 1981). Although, as we will see when we turn to campaigns in chapter 7, there has been concern for particular effects on some segments of the audience, in general the mass media focus on reaching large numbers of people simultaneously with the same message by the same means. In this sense, then, they share much with traditional approaches to public health. The general concern is to produce the greatest good in the greatest number. Accordingly, a fundamental indication of effect, or surrogate for effect, is a television program's rating, with higher ratings somewhat equivalent to dosage in the minds of advertisers.[2]

As we will see when we turn in more detail to communication campaigns, which often rely on mass media, it is often difficult to precisely control the frequency and sequencing of media exposure (Dijkstra, Buijtels,

& VanRaaij, 2005).[3] The media are less important than other sources for the socially integrated, but more important for the relatively socially isolated (Katz, Gurevitch, & Haas, 1973), who come to depend on the media for information, social comparisons, and modeling of coping processes (Aydin, Ball-Rokeach, & Reardon, 1991). The broader social trends relating to the new media and the Internet, and the resulting fragmentation of the audience, in some ways parallel the promise of genomics and personalized medicine.

EXPOSURE AND MEDIA EFFECTS

Mass media theory has been concerned fundamentally with when exposure, or a dose, will have an impact. Indeed, the earliest approaches are essentially simple metaphors that directly relate to dosage, at least in terms of an agent being directly administered to the audience. So you had the hypodermic needle model and also the magic bullet theory, with some parallels to the container metaphor. Audience members were thought to be relatively passive and defenseless.[4] Communication, in effect, could be shot into them (Schramm, 1972). This view of communication was embedded in the more general stimulus-response notions popular in psychological research in this time period (Rogers & Storey, 1987).

The underlying assumptions of bullet theory have been widely discredited within contemporary communication theory. It soon became clear that while messages might be delivered, the audience's interpretations of them might cause widely different reactions (Schramm, 1972), that the media only had limited effects. To many people this underlying approach, on its most primitive level, is also represented in the dosage metaphor. However, just as for communication, although somewhat more slowly, it has become clear that people's reactions to medicines and their feedback concerning them are critical to closing the loop on potential impacts.

SELECTIVE EXPOSURE

While there were some notable early successes, audiences could be remarkably resistant to mass media campaigns, especially those that did not correspond to the views of their immediate social networks (Katz & Lazersfeld, 1955; Rogers & Storey, 1987). So the simple stimulus response approaches represented by the magic bullet approach soon developed into a somewhat more sophisticated search for moderating variables or contexts in which media might have more powerful impacts. There developed a tendency among theorists of communication campaigns to cast "the audience as 'bad guys' who are hard to reach, obstinate, and recalcitrant" (Dervin, 1989, p. 73). The term "obstinate audience" was coined by Bauer (1972) in his classic research article detailing the active role audience members play in the processing of communication messages. In natural situations, Bauer contends, the audience selects what it will attend to. These selections often depend on interests, and the interests of audience members are reflected in the level of their knowledge and the strength of their convictions. While exposure is the first step to persuasion (McGuire, 1989), the audience members most likely to attend to messages are those already committed to them.

In a way, selective exposure, retention, and perception theories represent a form of self-medication determined by interest. Essentially, these theories argue that people play an active role in determining what therapeutic agents they will expose themselves to,[5] with individuals choosing media they are attuned to based on their viewpoint on particular issues, supporting their preexisting biases. So, media exposure often serves to maintain and reinforce existing beliefs (Berelson, Lazarsfeld, & McPhee, 1954). Thus people, in effect, determine their own dosages. Sears and Freedman (1967), in their classic review of this literature, suggest that things are somewhat more complicated than this simple assertion and that the magnitude of this effect is small. But they were writing in a time when there was not a proliferation of media choices, which makes it all the more likely in today's environment that selective exposure may play a major role in determining media effects. Another predictor of selective exposure is the perceived usefulness of the information, which provides a nice transition to uses and gratifications approaches, a subject we will return to in chapter 6.[6]

USES AND GRATIFICATIONS

The assumptions of uses and gratifications theory are particularly important for a renewed focus on receivers, which is implied in the dosage metaphor. Fundamentally, uses and gratifications theory suggests that individual receivers differentially select and use communication vehicles to gratify felt needs (Katz, Blumler, & Gurevitch, 1974; Katz, Gurevitch, & Haas, 1973; Rubin, 1986; Tan, 1985). Audiences are not passively waiting; rather they knowingly select channels on the strength of their perceived needs, and these needs ultimately determine a medium's impact (Lometti, Reeves, & Bybee, 1977). First, uses and gratifications assumes that media use is goal directed (Katz et al., 1973; Rubin, 1986; Tan, 1985), that the audience actively puts messages to use, and this moderates their effects (Katz et al., 1974). Second, it assumes receivers select differing media and content to fulfill felt needs

(Katz et al., 1973; Rubin, 1986; Tan, 1985). Third, uses and gratifications theory assumes that individuals initiate media selection (Katz et al., 1973; Rubin, 1986). Individuals will base their choices of channels, or delivery systems, in a way that will maximize the gratifications obtained, especially in relation to gratifications sought (Dobos, 1988). Fourth, there are multiple sources of needs satisfaction, and any one communication channel must compete with other channels for satisfaction of individual needs (Tan, 1985). Fifth, "people are aware of communication alternatives and select channels based on the normative images those channels are perceived to possess" (Perse & Courtright, 1993, p. 501).

Uses and gratifications theory, by suggesting that individuals will turn to specific media channels to fulfill specific cognitive or affective information needs, helps us to understand why individuals differentially expose themselves to channels and contents. So, people who are generally interested in health may become regular viewers of *The Dr. Oz Show* on the television when they have time in their afternoons. Uses and gratifications theory stresses the functions (and dysfunctions) that media serve for users. It also suggests that once gratifications are obtained, this reinforces beliefs that a particular source is gratifying, resulting in increased probability of future usage (Palmgreen, 1984). This closing of the loop is a crucial issue in the maintenance of proper doses of medicine as well. Perhaps the most telling theoretical weakness of the uses and gratifications approach is its failure to specify the initial motivating conditions for media usage (Rubin, 1986; Tan, 1985). The Comprehensive Model of Information Seeking (CMIS), which we turn to next, accomplishes this in specifying antecedent conditions for information seeking.

COMPREHENSIVE MODEL OF INFORMATION SEEKING

The CMIS, while growing out of many of the mass media approaches we have just discussed (Afifi, 2009), seeks to explain more generally how people will go about searching for answers to questions they may have.[7] My own struggles with securing cancer information provided the impetus for the development of this model. The CMIS has been empirically tested in a variety of cancer (J. D. Johnson, 1993b; J. D. Johnson & Meischke, 1993b) and organizational (J. D. Johnson et al., 1995) contexts. J. D. Johnson (2003) has systematically compared these two contexts and their implications for the CMIS. The CMIS focuses on the antecedents that explain why people become information seekers, the information carrier characteristics that shape how people go about looking for information, and the information seeking actions that reflect the nature of the search itself (see box 5.1 on *Lorenzo's Oil* for an application of the model to a concrete situation).

BOX 5.1.   THE CMIS AND *LORENZO'S OIL*

The film *Lorenzo's Oil* could be described as the perfect information seeking film, detailing as it does in a dramatic way the problems parents of children with exotic diseases encounter when they search for effective treatments.

The film focuses on dramatizing the actual case of Augusto and Michaela Odone and their son, Lorenzo, who contracts the genetically inherited disease of adrenoleukodystrophy (ALD). This is a particularly devastating disease that causes deterioration of the myelin sheath surrounding nerve cells, resulting in rapidly progressing incapacity if not arrested. At the time of their child's diagnosis, there was no known treatment for this orphan disease, which, because of its rarity, was not subject to intensive research efforts.

In terms of the antecedents of the CMIS, the Odones were very well-educated upper-middle-class professionals. They had rich social networks that often resulted in crucial weak ties that led them to clues to the ultimate answers they sought. They had no direct personal experience with this disease and were devastated by its genetic component since they had no knowledge of its appearing in Michaela's family in the past. This, in part, increased their drive to seek answers to this problem such that, since it had such salience, in very real ways it became their life. In terms of beliefs and the associated concept of self-efficacy, they never gave up hope that they had the skills to uncover answers and that information seeking for them was their only hope for coping with their child's illness.

The information characteristics of the CMIS are less explicitly covered in the dramatic narrative of *Lorenzo's Oil*, but it is clear that the Odones have a very sophisticated approach to information carriers. This is especially revealed in the utility that they saw in face-to-face conferences of leading experts.

What is unusual about their story, which also has much to say about the amount, frequency, and sequencing elements of dosage, is the incredible persistence of this family in their quest for information relating to uncovering potential treatments, which eventually resulted in the highly specialized oil that is the subject of the title of the film. While only arresting the progression of the disease in their child, this discovery helped many other children whose problems were identified soon enough. It also set the Odones on another quest to discover how myelin can be restored. They, then, embody many of the characteristics of the citizen scientist and hyperactive information seekers whose quest can be greatly facilitated by the Internet.

Antecedents

The antecedents of the CMIS include demographics, personal experience, salience, and beliefs. Information seeking can also be triggered by an individual's degree of direct, personal experience with the problem at hand. In the CMIS framework two personal relevance factors, salience and beliefs, are seen as the primary determinants in translating a perceived gap into an active search for information. Salience refers to the personal significance of information to the individual.

Acquiring more information and enhancing awareness can increase uncertainty and, relatedly, stress levels. As a result individuals often choose to reduce this uncomfortable state through processes associated with denial, inertia, and apathy. Individuals often deny the presence of disturbing information rather than confronting it. They do not want to know certain things, or they hope problems will just go away (Case et al., 2005).

Information seeking is also affected by various cultural factors, since all cultures develop rules that limit the sharing of information. Natural language is well suited for ambiguity and deception, and often concerns for politeness lead us to equivocate, dissemble, and tell others "white lies." We may be limited by polite discourse in the extent to which we can self-disclose personal information, as we saw in chapter 3. Conversely, others may be limited in the questions they feel they can ask us and the strategies they can pursue in seeking information. Fundamentally, individual attempts to establish relations with others for the purposes of sharing information must be accepted by the other, and utilitarian concerns for both the value of information and the social standing of individuals determine acceptance (Nebus, 2006).

Individuals' perception of the extent to which they can shape or control events will also have an impact on their level of awareness. For many individuals it does not make much sense to learn more about things over which they have no control, so the powerless tend not to seek information. Case et al. (2005) have articulated systematically why the avoidance of information may be very rational in particular situations where people have low self-efficacy or face threatening information (Ashford, Blatt, & VandeWalle, 2003). Often people do not have a sense of self-efficacy that they will be able to correctly interpret and react to any new information they are presented with. It may be perfectly rational then to avoid information when there is nothing one can do with the answers one may obtain. If the threat is extreme, or if any potential responses are not expected to be effective, then an attractive alternative is to ignore the threat entirely—to skip one's dosage, to not take one's medicine—which in turn promotes cognitive consistency (Case et al., 2005).

Information Carrier Factors

The information carrier factors contained in the CMIS are drawn from a model of Media Exposure and Appraisal (MEA) that has been tested on a variety of information carriers, including both sources and channels, and in a variety of cultural settings (J. D. Johnson, 1983, 1984a, 1984b, 1987; J. D.

Johnson & Oliveira, 1988). Following the MEA, the CMIS focuses on editorial tone, communication potential, and utility. In the CMIS characteristics are composed of editorial tone, which reflects an audience member's perception of credibility, while communication potential relates to issues of style and comprehensiveness.

Utility, in both the CMIS and MEA, relates the characteristics of a medium directly to the needs of an individual and shares much with the uses and gratifications perspective (Palmgreen, 1984). For example, is the information contained in the medium relevant, topical, and important for the individual's purposes?

Actions

Naturally there are several types of information seeking actions that can result from the impetus provided by the forgoing set of factors contained in the CMIS. For example, Lenz (1984) argues that search behavior can be characterized by its extent, or the number of activities carried out, which has two components: scope, the number of alternatives investigated, and depth, the number of dimensions of an alternative investigated. She also identifies the method of the search, or channel, as another major dimension of the search. J. D. Johnson (2009b), in discussing how people seek out information relating to work-life problems, has also specified actions individuals follow in their social networks in terms of seeking out opinion leaders, small world strategies, and transactive memory.

Since the development of the CMIS, Johnson et al. (2006) have become interested in the sequencing of information seeking, particularly in terms of the pathways people follow in obtaining answers to their questions. These pathways, in part, indicate the persistence of individuals, a critical issue for information seekers, who typically do not expend much effort in acquiring information. Pathways are also a way to operationalize sequencing, with potentially different outcomes for individuals depending on the pathways they follow to obtain answers to their questions. So, individuals who make the wrong choices initially, given the general lack of persistence, may prematurely end their search before they acquire the information they need.

Research on CMIS suggests it provides the "bare bones" of a causal structure, although the nature of the specific relationships contained in the model appears to be context dependent. Tests of CMIS in health situations suggests the model works best with authoritative channels, such as doctors, that are the object of intense, goal-directed searches (J. D. Johnson, 1993b; J. D. Johnson & Meischke, 1993b) and for rational, programmed tasks that are more proximate to the individual (J. D. Johnson et al., 1995).

DEPENDENCY

Partially in response to limited effects approaches, Sandra Ball-Rokeach and Melvyn DeFleur (1976) offered dependency theory to establish a set of conditions where mass media might have pronounced effects. First, they proposed that media's influence is based on its relationship to a number of other societal systems, suggesting a tripartite audience-media-society relationship. Second, they argued that media only has pronounced effects on individuals when they depend on it primarily or exclusively for information related to their need to understand their social world, to act meaningfully and effectively in that world, or to escape from daily problems and tensions. Box 5.2 on media fragmentation and public health details some contemporary manifestations of this theory. Third, this dependency is likely to increase in situations where the information is of increasing relevance because of conflict, change, or other factors in society.

BOX 5.2.   MEDIA FRAGMENTATION
AND PUBLIC HEALTH

Following the logic of dependency theory, the ever-growing fragmentation of media outlets and the widespread use of the Internet run the risk of significantly diluting the dose of any public health messages agencies might wish to distribute.

Historically the limited number of broadcast channels facilitated the work of public health agencies. They could talk to the general managers of the three television stations in town and, through them, get widespread diffusion of important messages. But this comfortable world has changed radically with the advent of the Internet and cable television stations. Now public health messages need to be distributed through scores, if not hundreds or even thousands, of channels to get the same reach that was so easy to achieve only a couple of decades ago.

This fragmentation has also played a role in the legitimation of very troubling phenomenon, such as the widespread resistance to vaccination on the part of some parents due to unfounded reports that it is linked to autism. This belief is supported by the websites and other media that these parents choose to attend to. Eventually the growing proportion of children who are not vaccinated will lead to fertile ground for emerging epidemics.

KNOWLEDGE GAP

The concepts of an "information gap" and the "information poor" have been advanced in recent years as important policy issues, generally in terms of their broad societal ramifications (Chen & Hernon, 1982; Dervin, 1980; Doctor, 1992; Siefert, Gerbner, & Fisher, 1989). There is a growing difference in exposure and access to information that reflects demographic classifications, such as socioeconomic status. A major impediment to health communication for some groups is a lack of necessary information-processing skills, some as fundamental as a lack of health literacy and lack of knowledge of the primary language in which most health matters are expressed (Freimuth, Stein, & Kean, 1989). Perhaps even more importantly, "informational have-nots" in many respects represent the average US citizen, not a small minority of the population (Dervin, 1989; Doctor, 1992), and these individuals risk becoming members of a permanent underclass. Only 12% of US adults have proficient health literacy, and this is particularly problematic among those older than 75, with only 1% of them proficient (US Department of Health and Human Services, 2010).

This has parallels in the increasing divisions in our health care system between the insured and uninsured. In response to these trends, governmental agencies are adopting policies to promote information equity among various segments of our society. This is especially true for rural populations, which have received special emphasis from federal policy makers in relation to telemedicine and, more recently, broadband.

The knowledge gap hypothesis (Tichenor, Donohue, & Olien, 1970) argues that over time gaps will increase, since more highly educated individuals assimilate new information faster from traditional mass media than more poorly educated ones; they also have more relevant social contacts, who are likely to discuss issues with them. In one form, this hypothesis suggests that these gaps are perpetual and that, ironically, agency efforts to disseminate information only increase the gaps existing in society, since the educated will assimilate the information more quickly and completely (Viswanath et al., 1993). In addition, access to technology and software is likely to be greater for privileged groups within our society.

While the knowledge gap has generally been supported in static studies, its exact dynamics over time are still subject to some debate (Freimuth, 1990; Viswanath et al., 1993). Gaps are smaller for topics that are of local interest, that do differentially interest certain groups (e.g., the performance capabilities of a Grand Cherokee versus a GMC Terrain), and that are couched in nontextbook terms (Freimuth, 1990).

Several underlying dynamics have been suggested for the existence and persistence of gaps. The deficit or individual blame bias suggests that information haves possess superior communication skills (e.g., reading, listening), a framework for understanding new information, and a greater range of social contacts. The difference position notes that among groups in our society many barriers exist to knowledge acquisition, including illiteracy (non-native-language speakers); "information ghettos," where there is primarily a one-way flow of information; exclusive within-group communication that further reinforces ignorance; and the often fatalistic cultures of disadvantaged groups.

It has been argued that the use of mass media can act to reduce gaps relating to issues that are of interest to normally disadvantaged groups (Freimuth, 1990; Freimuth, Stein, & Kean, 1989); furthermore, at some point the haves become satiated, and the poor can catch up (Dervin, 1980). Indeed, a recent study suggests that attention to health coverage reduces knowledge differences associated with differing levels of media coverage (Slater et al., 2009). Another way of stating this is to suggest that there are ceiling effects for some knowledge. So, simple messages (e.g., wear your seat belt) and finite knowledge of a particular event (e.g., Farah Fawcett died of anal cancer) increase the possibility for reduced gaps between audience members (Freimuth, 1990).

Inevitably, differential access to information produces differential participation rates in our society (Lievrouw, 1994). Classically our mass media infrastructure has produced information fields that are *informing*. They are geared to providing information they select that is then consumed by their audiences. Increasingly, information technologies offer the possibility of *involving* audience members through their interactive capabilities and enhanced possibilities for information seeking (Lievrouw, 1994).

It has been suggested that policy makers should strive to create information equity among different segments of our society as well as more globally (Siefert, Gerbner, & Fisher, 1989). One underlying reason for creating equity is that the wider the range of ideas available to individuals, the more likely it is that a plurality will gravitate toward the correct one.

Even if there is not a knowledge gap, there is a utilization gap. This utilization gap arises, in part, because some individuals are consciously deciding to decline membership in the information society (Fortner, 1995). Some people have just reached a saturation point; they cannot spend any more time communicating (Fortner, 1995); there may be an upper bound to the dosages they can receive.

We have always had among us Luddites who reject new technologies because they are socially and economically disadvantaged by them. We also have many individuals whom we typically don't like to talk about, who really don't want to know things, who are more interested in "vegging out" and being entertained (Fortner, 1995). While over and over again on a societal level we emphasize the need for individuals who will constantly grow and develop into perpetual learners, it must be acknowledged that some individuals would prefer a comfortable world where they do not need to change or expend the necessary effort to become healthy. So, we have the hyperwell, who have a very trendy approach to health fads and are constantly exercising, while the vast majority of the population becomes more unwell and obese.

The information revolution is contributing to the accelerating fragmentation of our culture (Fortner, 1995). This has led to considerable concern that individuals and organizations with resources and access will perpetuate (or even widen) gaps in information to preserve or enhance their power and economic advantages (Doctor, 1992; Lievrouw, 1994) or perpetuate unfounded beliefs such as those discussed in box 5.2 on public health.

SUMMARY AND COMMENTARY

Table 5.1 contains a summary of how the various mass media approaches relate to the dosage elements. Often these theories do not rigidly separate issues relating to amount and frequency. The bullet theory in its essence argued that only limited amounts of information, often in one-shot doses, are needed to change individuals. But this formulation soon ran into problems in empirical research, which led to more limited effects approaches, often characteristic of modern campaigns, to these issues. Looking at things from the other side, in terms of interest of audience members, selective exposure and uses and gratifications argue that the audience determines usage. In uses and gratifications and the CMIS individuals are essentially determining how useful they see the carrier to be, thus determining their own self-dosage. On the other hand, both dependency theories and knowledge gap approaches argue that larger structural features of the environment, primarily related to issues of access in one way or another, determine the amount and frequency of media use.

Sequencing is not a major issue in most of these approaches. Bullet theory perhaps most optimistically assumed more of a one-shot approach to the delivery of messages, almost equivalent to vaccination for smallpox. For the other theories, this issue is mostly implied or has limited discussion, although Johnson and his colleagues (J. D. Johnson et al., 2006) recently discussed issues of pathways that directly relate to sequencing. Knowledge gap approaches argue, however, that it is possible, after a long period of time, for audience members in different segments to converge on the same level of knowledge of particular issues.

By their very nature mass media approaches focus on a limited array of potential delivery systems. Modern approaches to mediated communication

Table 5.1. Comparing Mass Media Approaches and the Dosage Metaphor

			Mass Media Approaches			
Dosage Elements	Bullet Theory	Selective Exposure	Uses and Gratifications	CMIS Theory	Dependency	Knowledge Gap
Amount	Limited	Determined by interest	Self-medication	Information carrier factors	Increase in crisis	Determined by socioeconomics
Frequency	One shot	Determined by interest	Self-medication	Information carrier factors	Increase in crisis	Determined by socioeconomics
Sequencing	One shot	Implied	Implied	Pathways	Implied	Convergence
Delivery systems	Mass media	Determined by interest	Gratifications obtained	Characteristics	Presence of competitors	Differential access
Interactions	Simple explanations	Availability	Access	Rationality, authority	Relevance, other social systems	Deficits
Contraindications	Inoculated audience	Lack of alternatives	Lack of alternatives	Limited skill set	Alternative sources	Satiation, new or simple phenomenon
Dysfunctions	Naiveté	Fragmentation	Gluttony, bad foraging	Frustration, limited persistence	Third-party control	Disparities

open up a panoply of potential channels, including various forms of electronic, new media that often share characteristics with interpersonal channels, such as the Internet. Bullet theory assumed that the choice is up to the deliverer of a message. Selective exposure, uses and gratifications, and the CMIS each in their own way maintain that within the array of potential channels, people make choices depending on the medium's characteristics. Dependency theory and knowledge gap approaches suggest that the availability of various media is the critical issue.

Bullet theory approached these issues in a very simplistic way, with no allowance for interactive effects. Interestingly selective exposure and uses and gratifications treat larger societal issues of availability and access in terms of their interactions with potential mass media effects. J. D. Johnson (2009a) increasingly has focused on issues of rationality and related notions of authority in discussing the context in which the CMIS is most usefully applied. Knowledge gap approaches consider the issue of deficits in understanding as particularly important for determining the effects on different audience members of media messages.

Given the taken-for-granted status of mass media and the way they permeate our society, very little thought is given to whether or not they are contraindicated. Inoculation theory developed in response to bullet theory approaches, indicating when they might be contraindicated. Using media for persuasive attempts associated with rich, equivocal, complex problems also might be contraindicated (Fidler & Johnson, 1984). Simple problems, for which it is easy to become satiated with knowledge, reduce the possibility of knowledge gaps. The contraindications for the other theories, which, given the richness of our current media environment, are unlikely to pertain, primarily deal with the lack of alternative sources of information.

Administrative research, which is centrally concerned with dosage issues and associated with bullet theory, has increasingly been supplanted with critical theory that asks larger questions about societal impact. Each of these theories focuses on a different set of such societal concerns: fragmentation into separate interest groups for selective exposure, indulging in one's preferences for uses and gratifications, limited persistence in seeking information on even the most pressing issues for the CMIS, third-party manipulation for dependency theories, and marked disparities in exposure to needed information for knowledge gaps.

NOTES

1. Often the rationale for arguing for daily usage of newspapers is somewhat like that for vitamins: an apple a day keeps the doctor away.

2. It is interesting that a considerable proportion of basic texts on mass communications are based on numbers: the highest gross rating, the most popular movie, and so forth. These numbers become, in a very real way, a surrogate for impact, importance, and effect and content (Kent, 2001). On a fundamental level, why do advertisers and public relations folks spend millions to get exposure if it is not having an impact?

3. Some "people-meter-type" systems attempt to continuously record attention to what people are watching.

4. When it turned out that audience members were not quite so passive, inoculation theory, which explained resistance based on biological analogy, was promulgated (McGuire, 1961). Essentially this theory, drawing on a classic biological metaphor, suggests that people can build up resistance to future persuasion attempts by being exposed to weakened examples of future opposing messages, in much the way vaccines function (Littlejohn & Foss, 2011). This also provides them with practice in counterarguing. Potential threats motivate receivers to strengthen their attitudes, thus protecting them against future attacks, with sequencing issues like delay also potentially important (Banas & Rains, 2010). In a recent attempt to expand inoculation theory metaphor, M. L. M. Wood (2007) suggested that, in addition to operating on subjects who held the preferred attitude, it could be extended to those more neutral or even opposed.

5. This has interesting parallels with the routes to persuasion suggested in the Elaboration Likelihood Model, which suggests under what conditions messages are most likely to have direct or indirect impacts, with central processing occurring when one is motivated and able to carefully evaluate the arguments and to scrutinize the quality of messages (Petty & Cacioppo, 1986).

6. However, one recent study suggests a more nuanced view of the phenomenon for online information. It suggests, at least for political matters, that while people seek out information consistent with their views, this does not mean they do not attend to messages opposing them, suggesting separate processes for these two different types of information (Garrett, 2009).

7. This is somewhat akin to the process of individuals seeking medications for what ails them. In general, people who go through a great deal of trouble to attain something value it more highly; the scarcer a piece of information is, the more likely it is to be persuasive (Cialdini, 2001).

FURTHER READINGS

Ball-Rokeach, S. J., & DeFleur, M. L. (1976). A dependency model of mass media effects. *Communication Research, 1*, 3–21.
    Specified when the tripartite media-audience-society relationship was most likely to produce media effects. In essence, the media is more likely to have pronounced impacts the more dependent the latter two members of this relationship are when there are few alternatives for information and there is rapid social change.

Johnson, J. D., & Case, D. O. (2012). *Health information seeking*. New York: Peter Lang.

A detailed treatment of health information seeking organized around the Comprehensive Model of Information Seeking. It also systematically compares the CMIS to other models of information seeking.

Slater, M. D. (2004). Operationalizing and analyzing exposure: The foundation of media effects research. *Journalism and Mass Communication Quarterly, 81*, 168–183.

Established a framework for his later work at Ohio State University with various colleagues on updating the selective exposure literature. Given the centrality of exposure to most theories of mass communication and communication campaigns, this article details operationalizations and analysis strategies that would advance mass media research.

Tichenor, P. J., Donohue, G. A., & Olien, C. N. (1970). Mass media and differential growth in knowledge. *Public Opinion Quarterly, 34*, 158–170.

The classic, seminal article on the knowledge gap.

· 6 ·

Diffusion and Dissemination

Designing for diffusion means taking additional steps early in the process of creating an innovation to increase its chances of being noticed, positively perceived, accessed and tried, adopted and implemented and thus, successfully crossing the research-to-practice chasm (J. W. Dearing & Kreuter, 2010, p. S100, italics in original).

$\mathcal{O}$ne of the most compelling uses of the dosage metaphor comes in its application to problems of change, which will be the focus of the next two chapters. There also is no more compelling issue related to health. Much morbidity and mortality are associated with an individual's unwillingness to adopt appropriate health behaviors, a topic we will return to in chapter 7, when we turn to communication campaigns and other more mass media–oriented efforts to impact publics. Our health care institutions and practitioners have also often been unwilling to adopt more appropriate approaches to treatment, which has led to an increased interest on the part of policy makers in clinical and translational science, which is the focus of this chapter.

CLINICAL AND TRANSLATIONAL SCIENCE

The transfer of ideas, often referred to as diffusion or dissemination, has drawn increased attention over the last decade.[1] One of the most exciting recent developments in change research is the growing focus of the National Institutes of Health (2006), in part responding to congressional pressure, on translational and dissemination research. The central issue for policy makers is that, while there has been an explosion of knowledge in the laboratory, very little gets translated into clinical practice, and even less is widely and faithfully implemented (Bradley et al., 2004). So, what we know is not changing what we do, producing troubling returns on investment for research. This is part of a more widespread problem that is generic to most organizations (Ansari, Fiss, & Zajac, 2010), with effective practices developed in one division seldom spreading to another (J. W. Dearing, 2006; Szulanski, 2003).

The evidence for widespread dissemination of effective practices is discouraging in health (L. A. Green & Seifert, 2005; Klesges et al., 2005; Orleans, 2005) and more general managerial settings (Szulanski, 2003). It has been suggested that it takes an average of 17 years for a fraction of efficacious treatments to move into practice (Glasgow, Marcus, et al., 2004). This is especially worrying because of clinicians' knowledge deterioration after they graduate (West et al., 1999). Much research has been done over the years, and very expensive interventions developed, that has little chance of actually being implemented in practice (Glasgow, Klesges, et al., 2004; J. D. Johnson, 2005; Klesges et al., 2005), in part because of the lack of understanding of the dosage required.

An interesting exemplar of an approach to these issues for health behavior interventions is the RE-AIM Framework developed by Glasgow and his colleagues (Glasgow, Klesges, et al., 2004; Glasgow, Lichtenstein, & Marcus, 2003; Glasgow, Marcus, et al., 2004; Glasgow, Vogt, & Boles, 1999; L. W. Green & Glasgow, 2006; Klesges et al., 2005) (http://www.re-aim.org). Essentially this approach proposes that translation and public health impact are best evaluated along the following five dimensions: reach into target population, efficacy or effectiveness, adoption, implementation, and maintenance. This constitutes a relatively long-linked chain with probabilities of success at each stage relatively slight, suggesting that the ultimate end result is unlikely to be successful (Glasgow, Vogt, & Boles, 1999).

There seems to be an implicit assumption in most settings that if you build it they will come, that if you make a better mousetrap, it will be widely adopted. Thus, subsequent diffusion of ideas gets little attention (and fewer resources) (Glasgow, Marcus, et al., 2004). No one, especially the original researchers, has a clear responsibility for dissemination (Glasgow, Marcus, et al., 2004; J. D. Johnson, 2005), and little formal research, at least in health care settings, has focused on implementation (Oldenburg et al., 1999), whose costs may outweigh the benefits of the intervention (Grimshaw et al., 2004). There is often considerable inertia in social settings; resistance to new ideas; concern over diminishment of one's autonomy, personal judgment, and creativity associated with professions; and an unwillingness to adopt good ideas developed by others since that often reduces one's own status (think of researchers in academe). Especially important in medical settings, particularly private practice, is push-back from patients (Freeman & Sweeney, 2001).

The National Institutes of Health initiatives fit in with a growing, more general interest in translation science, which focuses on "how evidence-based practices, programs, and policies can best be communicated for adaptation by practitioners in a societal sector for the benefit of their constituents" (J. W. Dearing, 2006, p. 3). This is more specialized than the classic diffusion study since it focuses on evidence-based practices, which require fidelity in their implementation (see box 6.1); it is also predictive and interventionist, targets practitioners, and draws on a wide array of disciplines to encourage spread (J. W. Dearing, 2006).

BOX 6.1. FIDELITY

> The most commonly used measures of fidelity are adherence to the program, dose (amount of the program delivered), quality of program delivery, and participant reaction or acceptance. . . . To make programs more acceptable, adaptability is often built in, yet this adaptability makes fidelity more difficult to achieve (Rohrbach et al., 2006, pp. 308).

Because of the focus on evidence-based practices, an important element of diffusion research is a focus on fidelity (Glasgow, Klesges, et al., 2004), since seldom are interventions adopted or implemented exactly as they were originally tested (L. W. Green & Glasgow, 2006),[2] which plays havoc with evidence-based approaches. Effect fidelity relates to the ability of an intervention to achieve the same effects across multiple contexts. This directly relates to the external validity of tests of a program. Implementation fidelity relates to the exact replication of a program across multiple settings (J. W. Dearing, 2006). This aspect of fidelity directly conflicts with reinvention and the exercise of creativity and professional judgment by the adopting unit; it also fails to recognize that highly motivated, even dogmatic recipients are likely to change the nature of interventions in their search for efficacious practices (Szulanski, 2003).

Some modifications may be absolutely essential for translating a practice to a new context. The question is one of balance and whether or not the core, the purity of the therapeutic agent if you will, of what worked in the intervention, is preserved (J. W. Dearing & Kreuter, 2010; L. W. Green & Glasgow, 2006). This dynamic is somewhat evocative of physicians tempering the recommended dosages in chemotherapy, where often patients find the recommended dosages intolerable for a number of reasons (Mukherjee, 2010). Of course, all this is further complicated by best practices often being a moving target (Szulanski, 2003). Some have suggested that working on basic contextual factors (e.g., assuring appropriate levels of training and resources), while preserving the intervention, may be the best approach (Elliott & Mihalic, 2004).

TRANSFER OF KNOWLEDGE

Theories of change often appeal to metaphors, so we have: learning systems (Marshak, 1996), hooks, things in one's own experience that one can attach new knowledge to in Leonard's (2006) terms, or stickiness in Szulanski's (1996, 2003) terms, evoking images of immobility, inertness, inimitability, and resistance to change. Stickiness focuses on the general failure of best practices to spread within an organization (Szulanski, 2003), which turns our attention to the properties of communication networks.

Network analysis is a key source of concepts that enrich our understanding of dosage within communication research, particularly for diffusion of innovation research. An important general property of a network link is its strength, with the frequency of communication used to indicate the strength of a link (Richards, 1985). The strength of weak ties, a critical concept related to diffusion, directly relates to the amount and frequency elements of the dosage metaphor. It has been associated with the flow of information and the transfer of knowledge and by definition is removed from stronger social bonds.

Information from weak ties is useful precisely because it comes from infrequent or weak contacts. Strong contacts are likely to be people with whom there is a constant sharing of the same information; as a result individuals within cohesive social groups have come to have the same information base. However, information from outside this base gives unique perspectives and, in some instances, strategic advantages over competitors in a person's immediate network.

Weak ties provide critical informational support because they transcend the limitations of our strong ties and because, as often happens, our strong ties can be disrupted or unavailable. Thus weak ties may be useful for discussing things you do not want to reveal to your close associates, providing a place for an individual to experiment, extending access to information, promoting social comparison, and fostering a sense of community (Adelman, Parks, & Albrecht, 1987). They are also essential to creativity (see box 6.2).

All of this again suggests the nature of match, the importance of measured dosages. While strong direct ties have compelling advantages for influence, the transfer of tacit knowledge, and potential spillover effects for resource sharing, they are costly to maintain and redundant, especially so in the opportunity costs of reducing the number of weak ties we might have. On the other hand, indirect ties allow us to experiment and scan our environment widely for information, but these links have difficulty transferring that knowledge.

BOX 6.2. CREATIVITY

Over the last decade a clear understanding has emerged in the network literature of the forces that help shape creativity. There is an underlying nonlinear, inverted, U-shaped element to creative work, with some contact (often through small world processes and weak ties) necessary for stimulation, but too much contact results in conformity pressures that dampen creativity (Uzzi & Spiro, 2005).

Paradoxically the more people communicate, the more they converge on a common attitude, the less creative they are. However, while cohesion limits creativity, it aids the spread and transfer of knowledge. Thus, the same forces that may limit creativity may facilitate the implementation of innovations.

All of this suggests the delicate temporal challenges (and the sequencing of doses) for those who wish to maintain diversity, in part to enhance creative responses to a changing world and the importance of processes that lead to uniformity of attitudes and behaviors necessary for implementation (Balkundi & Harrison, 2006) and the ultimate translation of ideas into clinical and translational science applications.

SOCIAL CONTAGION

Social contagion refers to the processes by which ideas spread in social systems and often draws directly from health perspectives on the spread of diseases. Cohesion and structural equivalence views of social contagion have emerged as alternative theoretic frames for the understanding of diffusion and dissemination. They essentially represent alternative views as to whether direct communication or forces related to competition, respectively, are the major motive forces within social systems. (See box 6.3.) Cohesion perspectives fit clearly into the "communication metamyth" perspective that more is necessarily better, while structural equivalence perspectives suggest that in some circumstances no direct communication contacts are necessary, the most radical minimalist position.

Change is often assumed to be a cognitive process involving awareness, attitudes, and beliefs.[3] So social influence processes become critical for understanding the underlying dynamics and mechanisms of change (McGrath & Krackhardt, 2003). Media effects are also moderated by the social context of individuals, as we will discuss in more detail in chapter 7. Increasingly, studies are finding relationships between social networks and a variety of health-related issues, with one-study finding a linear, monotonic relationship between frequency of discussing alcohol in college networks and drinking behaviors (Dorsey, Scherer, & Real, 1999). In addition, over the last several years a major debate has developed about whether direct communication or forces related to competition are the major motive forces for innovation adoption, a traditional focus of campaigns. If competitors adopt an innovation and it is successful, this will put another individual at a competitive disadvantage. So, the other has an incentive to adopt an innovation. Thus, individuals will adopt innovations when a structurally similar alter does, even if they are not in direct communication contact, a key perspective in a minimalist approach to dosage issues.

A cohesion perspective is implicit in most communication approaches to campaigns, which we will discuss in more detail in the next chapter, suggesting that direct communication results in changes in the individual that result in the adoption of innovations. Enthusiastic supporters of an innovation may directly communicate with members who were not involved in its development. This enthusiasm is contagious, and the members decide to adopt the innovation because of the credibility and persuasiveness of innovation champions.

Both cohesion and structural equivalence approaches to social contagion have been linked to diffusion and dissemination, with the former the traditional approach and the latter offering new insights. More recently it has been argued that they can have complementary effects on knowledge transfer, with cohesion easing it by reducing competitive impediments and tie strength impacting the transfer of tacit knowledge (Reagans & McEvily, 2003). This suggests that individuals' information fields and (in a more encompassing sense) their structurally equivalent positions within networks may be the primary determinants of the diffusion of innovations. (See box 6.3 for a more complete discussion.)

Attitude formation and related cohesion processes in human communication networks have long been a crucial concern in the social sciences generally. Indeed, a number of mathematical models in essence argue, from a cohesion perspective, that greater amounts (or doses) of communication result in greater attitude similarities within networks. These discrepancy models of attitude change have received empirical support in a number of contexts (Danes, Hunter, & Woelfel, 1978; Goldberg, 1954; Zimbardo, 1960) and essentially hypothesize that attitude change is a function of the distance between initial attitudes and the rate of contact between any two communicators, a more formal expression of cohesion arguments.

For noncontroversial change, the key structural issue is how to promote the widespread, rapid communication of the underlying notions using structural leverage (McGrath & Krackhardt, 2003). Interestingly, McGrath and Krackhardt (2003) also argue that for controversial changes, to reduce the probability of backlash and resulting counterinfluence attempts, it is better to let change unfold, demonstrating its effectiveness, by piloting it at the periphery, before attempting broader dissemination (McGrath & Krackhardt, 2003).

BOX 6.3.   DIFFUSION OF TETRACYCLINE

One of the classic research studies in the social sciences is that by Coleman and his colleagues (Coleman, Katz & Menzel, 1957) that focused on the diffusion of an innovation among physicians. This study has been reexamined periodically with new methods and conceptions of key concepts and has become one of the touchstones of the innovation literature. It focused on the diffusion of a new drug through the network of interpersonal relationships among physicians in four cities in the Midwest. Doctors who were more oriented to their professions used the drug earlier, when there was still some uncertainty about its adoption, than those who were more patient oriented. More socially integrated doctors showed an accelerating gap over time in their adoptions. Later adopters appear to be eventually influenced by such sources as detail men representing pharmaceutical companies, ads, journal articles, and so on. But in all cases elements of the dosage metaphor were critical to the analysis particularly of sequencing, frequency, amount, and delivery systems.

Thirty years later, with advancements in research methods and a critical theoretic distinction, Ron Burt (1987) reanalyzed these classic findings. He suggested that while the original study focused on the cohesive effects of direct communication contacts, it was actually competitive forces associated with the similar structural positioning, structural equivalence, that best explained the research findings. Both of these processes relate to the more encompassing problem of social contagion, which seeks to explain the diffusion of innovations in social systems under conditions of uncertainty. Generally Burt suggests that contagion was not the major influence on adoption (personal preferences were) and that when it was a factor, physicians were quick to adopt because they feared that other physicians would gain a competitive advantage (many were in private practice) over them since patient outcomes would improve so dramatically. So, physicians who were similarly positioned in the social structure appeared to adopt during the same time period.

Additional analysis of the classic Coleman, Katz, and Menzel (1957) tetracycline study, a primary early source of support for cohesion perspectives, suggests that marketing efforts by drug companies were the primary sources of influence, and cohesion actually had very little impact (Van den Bulte & Lillien, 2001), reinforcing the importance of mass media as well as interpersonal influence (T. Valente, 2006).

One major limiting condition to these processes is the amount of information that an individual already possesses relating to a particular attitude. Woelfel et al. (1980) argued that the greater the amount of information previously communicated to an individual, the less the likelihood that future messages can induce attitude change. This finding is also supported in a meta-analysis of US health communication campaigns, which stresses the importance for achieving pronounced campaign effects of presenting new information (L. B. Snyder & Hamilton, 2002). Huckfeldt, Johnson, and Sprague (2004), while recognizing the inertial, autoregressive force of an individual's existing information base, also suggest that an individual's positioning in low-density networks with ties to others who share their opinions will slow social change.

In organizations individuals within different units (e.g., administration, nursing) will come to adopt unique perspectives often associated with their functions (Lawrence & Lorsch, 1967) and their professions. It might be expected that if there were enough ties present between groups, then a whole organization network would eventually come to reflect a common position on a particular attitude (Abelson, 1964; French, 1956; Huckfeldt, Johnson, and Sprague 2004), a major promise of the interprofessional training we focused on in chapter 4. However, recognizing the openness of organizations to other institutions within the society (e.g., professional associations) and the mass media, it is unlikely that any organization will be isolated enough for the people within it to come to convergence (M. Taylor, 1968).

CRITICAL MASS AND THRESHOLD

> What we really need as a collective is evidence about the doing of *less*: minimum "good enough" interventions that not only achieve acceptable thresholds of desired outcomes, but outperform push-based strategies (J. W. Dearing & Kreuter, 2010, p. 102, italics in original).

Network simulations have examined how a few simple interaction rules result in the development of self-organizing systems. So, the susceptibility of a node to infection (usually a disease, but it could also be a new idea) spreads through direct contact with others, represented by threshold rules and how connected the system is, and can result in information cascades (Watts, 2003). T. W. Valente (1995) sought to explain the classic S-curve finding in diffusion research that after a slow building of early adopters, suddenly there is a rush to adopt. Threshold models suggest that people engage in behaviors when a sufficient proportion of others do, with individual thresholds varying. These variations result in the classic distributions of roles from early to late adopters in classic S-curve depictions of innovation adoption.

These thresholds also play a critical role in information cascades, more familiarly known as tipping points. The more heterogeneous a network is, the greater the unique information each link contains, the more susceptible it is to cascades (Watts, 2002). Individuals like opinion leaders, who are in network positions (e.g., liaisons) that expose them to more information earlier, are more likely to be earlier adopters (T. W. Valente, 1995). This also relates to box 6.3.

Critical mass represents the number of individuals needed before an innovation is likely to spread to others. One problem for the diffusion of communication technologies is that a certain number of users are needed to make them useful, a key factor in the adoption of social networking technologies like Twitter.

These two factors interact. Once an individual adopts an innovation, it lowers the thresholds of others because of decreased risk. The more individuals who adopt, the lower the risk, leading to a snowball effect (Watts, 2002).

IMPLEMENTATION

Metaphors should not be seen as a means for sugarcoating bitter pills (Armenakis & Bedeian, 1992, p. 297).

Successful implementation of an innovation, once it is disseminated, can be conceived of as routinization, incorporation, and stabilization in health practices: "The bottom line is implementation (including its institutionalization), and not just the adoption decision" (Rogers & Adhikayra, 1979, p. 79). Perhaps because of the operational nature of the processes associated with implementation, provocative metaphors are less in evidence at this stage, and those that are used often contain some element of resistance, such as the lead quote in this section, but the research that has been done has implicit relations to the dosage metaphor.

Communication plays a key role in overcoming resistance in part by reducing uncertainty. Complexity and risk are elements of uncertainty that are crucial to the ultimate implementation of innovations as detailed in box 6.4. The reduction of uncertainty inherent in communication can decrease resistance to innovations. Social contexts of relatively dense ties with redundant others can inhibit creativity and often lead to resistance, but they also build trust and cooperation while aiding tacit transfer of knowledge and influence attempts related to innovation implementation. In more decentralized environments and those with a large number of professionals associated with health care, messages from a wide range of sources may actually be more effective and less costly for an organization than exclusively relying on a top-down approach to innovation (Leonard-Barton & Deschamps, 1988).

BOX 6.4.   INFLUENCE AND
INNOVATION IMPLEMENTATION

Fidler and Johnson (1984) described systematically the consequences of using various types of influence processes in innovation implementation. Drawing on the classic framework of French and Raven (1959), they detailed the relatively high communication costs of the use of sanction and persuasion and the low costs of using legitimate and referent power. Different levels of involvement are related to the influence represented by persuasion, expert, and referent power, with the lower levels of involvement related to sanction and legitimate power. Expert power represents some special problems for the person exercising it. If every detail of an expert's thought process must be explained, especially in situations of high tacit knowledge, then very high communication costs are entailed. But if just a conclusion is needed, then its costs may be as low as those of legitimate power.

Complexity also affects innovation involvement, with some types of power potentially contraindicated. For example, the more facets to an innovation, the more actions that have to be rewarded and, somewhat relatedly, the greater the volume of information needed to persuade. The high communication costs of persuasion and sanction and also, in this case, expert power increase almost exponentially with greater complexity; however, the communication costs of other types of power increase more linearly because the invocation of these types of power is inherent in the messages concerning the innovation (Fidler & Johnson, 1984).

Generally, persuasive strategies have been found to be the most effective means of ensuring implementation, especially highly risky ones.[4] Effective persuasion can best overcome resistance attributable both to lack of understanding and to fear; in addition, the use of persuasion results in a higher level of involvement.

For informal channels, persuasion, or influence, is the primary means available to secure participation in an innovation. In utilizing persuasion an individual communicates evidence, arguments, and a rationale advocating acceptance, with organizational efforts very similar to the campaigns discussed in the next chapter. Since innovations within large organizations generally are initiated by an idea generator who must convince others to participate (Galbraith, 1982), the willingness to participate in innovations is a critical outcome of communication. Since effective persuasion results in greater participation in the implementation of innovations, it usually entails less resistance to the eventual implementation of innovations as well, and it is more likely to ensure active involvement. There is a critical difference between effective communication, where each party understands the other, and persuasive communication, where one of them changes his or her opinion as a result of communication (Huckfeldt, Johnson, & Sprague, 2004).

As box 6.4 details, complexity and perceived risk interact with types of power to determine the communication costs associated with their implementation. This introduces notions of the interaction of a number of therapeutic agents to produce desired impacts and the possibility that in certain circumstances innovation implementation is contraindicated.

SUMMARY

Returning to the problem of clinical and translational science as our touchstone, amount is a critical ingredient of most network analysis approaches to the transfer of ideas in social systems, with the central concept of the strength of weak ties suggesting innovations are more likely to flow from those people with whom we have little contact. So, medical innovations are more likely to spread through detail people representing drug companies or chance encounters with other medical professionals (see table 6.1). Conversely, for implementation, cohesion approaches to contagion argue that significant amounts of communication are needed in part because of the difficulties involved in communicating tacit information. So, implementation may be more likely to occur within an institution like a hospital. Amount is also central for threshold and critical mass approaches with substantial proportions needed for successful adoption.

Frequency is somewhat less clearly specified. Strength of weak ties entails infrequent communication with the other, with links that can decay very rapidly (Burt, 2002). Frequency of contact can also be associated with thresholds. Interestingly, for structural equivalence approaches to communication, very minimal amounts of communication may be needed.

In threshold/critical mass approaches, a certain level must be attained before they sequence to widespread "infection." Redundancy and repetition are elements of approaches to cohesion; following up on what you find from your weak ties with strong ones is important for the ultimate implementation of innovations (J. W. Dearing & Kreuter, 2010).

In general, innovation approaches put a premium on interpersonal contacts because of their ability to directly spread information through persuasion. However, as box 6.3 suggests, sometimes the advantages of an innovation are so compelling that mediated channels can also be successful delivery systems.

These approaches do not offer detailed conceptualization of interaction, contraindications, and dysfunctions. The more embedded people are in their social environment, the more pronounced conforming effects are going to be, and the less the likelihood of strength-of-weak-ties impacts. However, if context doesn't provide support and access to people motivated to help, then

Table 6.1. Comparing Diffusion Approaches and the Dosage Metaphor

| | Diffusion Approach | | |
Dosage Elements	Transfer	Social Contagion	Threshold/Critical Mass	Implementation
Amount	Minimal	High for cohesion	Critical levels	Contingent
Frequency	Episodic	Low for structural equivalence	Critical levels	Match
Sequencing	Follow-up	Repetition for cohesion	Staging	After adoption
Delivery systems	Relationships	Links for cohesion	Links	Various
Interactions	Density, embeddedness	Information fields	Heterogeneity	Cohesion
Contraindications	Motivation, access	Resistance	Risk	Low cohesion
Dysfunctions	Conformity	Lack of control	Innovation failure	Resistance

somebody may be impelled to seek out weak ties. For threshold and critical mass approaches, the level of perceived risk may eventually lead to innovation failure unless there are compensating incentives offered, such as those the US government is using to leverage the adoption of electronic health records.

NOTES

1. Translation itself is, of course, a metaphor (B. Johnson & Hagstrom, 2005).

2. Interestingly Ansari, Fiss, & Zajac (2010) specifically label one of their four dimensions of practice variability and adoption "low dosage" adoption, where the practice is faithful to prior work.

3. A classic problem in literature in this area relates to the degree and pervasiveness of organizational change embodied in any one effort. At one extreme, one might have a slight change in one organizational process, say different paper for reproducing documents, that impacts very little else; on the other extreme might be an encompassing change in an organization's structure and climate, say moving from a hierarchical framework to a truly virtual, decentralized organization. Needless to say, this type of change is very disruptive and very difficult to pull off, in part because of the forces of inertia reinforced by the routines embodied in structure, but also because of the seemingly inevitable (and often rapid) development of centralized, differentiated structures. It also evokes the classic knowledge transfer paradox, since fundamental change requires a certain level of tacit knowledge to implement, while at the same time introducing a significant learning problem (Tenkasi & Chesmore, 2003).

4. J. D. Johnson (1990) tested a model of the effects of persuasiveness, salience, and uncertainty on participation in innovations. This research focused on the role of informal communication channels as delivery systems for influence attempts related to a new component of an existing program. It examined the initial stages of the development of innovations at lower levels in an organization. The communication channel typically used in this phase is primarily interpersonal, and these subformal channels reflect the informal authority structure of an organization (Downs, 1967). Typically these more personal channels are more likely to be effective, since they meet the specific needs and questions of the receivers because of the immediacy of feedback and the situation specificity of the channel. As a result there is an inherent reduction of uncertainty involved in the use of these channels, since they lead to increased understanding of a proposed innovation, which may in part account for the somewhat more moderate impact of uncertainty in the model. J. D. Johnson's (1990) model was tested on data gathered from a large financial institution, and the results suggested that the classic communicative variable of persuasion had a paramount impact on participation, reinforcing the notion that communication is central to innovative processes within organizations.

FURTHER READINGS

Abelson, R. P. (1964). Mathematical models of the distribution of attitudes under controversy. In N. Frederiksen & H. Gulliksen (Eds.), *Contributions to mathematical psychology* (pp. 141–164). New York: Holt, Rinehart, and Winston.

A beautiful mathematical model describing how a simple model of discrepancies in initial attitudes between members of a network can eventually converge on a common attitude as a function of the amount of communication and similarities of contacts.

Burt, R. S. (1987). Social contagion and innovation: Cohesion versus structural equivalence. *American Journal of Sociology, 92*, 1287–1335.

A reexamination of the classic tetracycline study contrasting two classic explanations for social contagion: cohesion and structural equivalence.

Coleman, J., Katz, E., & Menzel, H. (1957). The diffusion of an innovation among physicians. *Sociometry, 20*, 253–270.

Seminal early study focusing on the role of communication networks in the diffusion of medical innovations.

Rogers, E. M. (2003). *The diffusion of innovations* (5th ed.). New York: Free Press.

One of the most frequently cited works in the history of the social sciences. Near encyclopedic coverage of innovations in a variety of settings.

Szulanski, G. (1996). Exploring internal stickiness: Impediments to the transfer of best practice within the firm. *Strategic Management Journal, 17*, 27–43.

Highly cited work describing the difficulty in transferring knowledge related to best practices within firms. In effect, transfer is impeded by a number of factors classically associated with elements of communication models, including characteristics of the source, the receiver, and the context in which they are embedded.

· 7 ·

Change

Exposure is a necessary, but not a sufficient, condition for change in the target population (L. B. Snyder & Hamilton, 2002, p. 360).

What is the impact of various quantities of campaign messages? Research should examine (a) the minimum volume of stimuli needed to achieve meaningful effects on key outcomes and (b) the quantitative point of diminishing returns from larger volumes (Salmon & Atkin, 2003, p. 467).

Rather than relying on a handful of incentives, it is advantageous to use multiple appeals across a series of messages in a campaign to influence different segments of the target audience (especially in media channels where precise targeting is difficult) and too provide several reasons for an individual to comply (Salmon & Atkin, 2003, p. 457).

In this chapter we will describe the traditional approach to administrative communication that most clearly encapsulates the dosage metaphor—the work of various professionals attempting to achieve a clearly specified change in members of an audience, especially at a group level, during a limited period of time with communication campaigns (Salmon & Atkin, 2003). This is the most scientifically advanced area of dosage research in communication (at least in terms of quantitative approaches) (Hornik, 2002a; Noar, Palmgreen, & Zimmerman, 2009) because of the work of people in advertising, marketing, and public relations, but it is often very proprietary as a result.[1]

This makes the work of those involved in well-funded health communication campaigns all the more important for public access to scientific findings (Noar, 2006). These campaigns often adopt a dose-response perspective, arguing that those with greater exposure to campaign messages are more likely to adopt behavioral changes (Noar, Palmgreen, & Zimmerman, 2009). In part because the desired outcome and the therapeutic agent are so clear, traditionally these professionals have thought of these processes in terms of a one-way, top-down flow of communication. They have relied on the mass media to reach large numbers of people efficiently in their campaigns (e.g., increasing mammography screening). These authoritative dicta and the lack of interactivity in the communication channel, or delivery system, were meant as much to discourage dialogue as to stimulate it. As we have seen, many approaches and assumptions of traditional media research were often implicit in this approach. Before we turn to campaigns, however, a review of the behavioral science theories that underlie them is in order.

BEHAVIORAL SCIENCE APPROACHES

Given its pragmatic significance, considerable theoretical and empirical work has been devoted to the development of models associated with campaigns; for example, in the Theory of Reasoned Action (Ajzen, 1985, 1987; Ajzen & Fishbein, 1980; Fishbein & Ajzen, 1975), a person's commitment to engage in the target behavior is conceptualized as a "behavioral intention." These models have been systematically compared to each other, with often conflicting findings (e.g., Hill, Gardner, & Rassaby, 1985; Mullen, Hersey, & Iverson, 1987; Seibold & Roper, 1979). Here we will focus on those that have been most clearly aligned with the dosage metaphor.

Health Belief Model

Increasingly, illness and disease are being attributed, in part, to individuals' lifestyles and their ability (or willingness) to change certain health behaviors. This is reflected in a growing body of research on disease prevention that has focused on strategies for behavior change. Historically one theoretical framework that has been used extensively to explain and predict preventive health behaviors is the Health Belief Model (HBM), a social-psychological model based on value-expectancy theory, which, in part, grew out of the recognition of the high levels of noncompliance with medical advice we discussed in chapter 3 (Becker & Rosenstock, 1984). In general, it argues that people pursue positive outcomes and avoid negative ones (Meischke, 1991). Although this model incorporates many variables, scholars have generally tested only a few in any one investigation. The HBM has been the focus of intensive research, although it has primarily been examined in the context of preventive health behavior (Nemcek, 1990). For example, the HBM framework has been used to investigate breast cancer prevention behaviors such as breast self-examinations (Champion, 1985; Massey, 1986; Sheppard et al., 1990) and mammography screening (Calnan, 1984; Rimer et al., 1988). Its major relationships have received support across a range of studies, though the level of variance accounted for is relatively low (Calnan, 1984; Champion, 1987).

The variables contained in the HBM are drawn from the work of Lewin and other social psychologists (Kegeles, 1980; Mikhail, 1981). The HBM also shares certain similarities with uses and gratifications theory, a theory of media usage we discussed in chapter 5, which specifies the social environment, demographics, group affiliations, and personality characteristics as background factors (Tan, 1985).

The HBM includes seven major factors hypothesized to influence health behavior: background characteristics, knowledge/attitudes/beliefs, social/group norms, barriers to action, cues to action, readiness/behavioral intentions, and outcome behaviors (Becker et al., 1977; Becker & Rosenstock, 1989; Cummings, Becker, & Maile, 1980; Rosenstock, 1974). The HBM suggests that individuals will take preventive health actions when they perceive themselves to be susceptible to a disease, when the disease is perceived as a serious illness, and when the benefits to undertaking the recommended health behavior outweigh the barriers (Janz & Becker, 1984; Rosenstock, 1974). Some stimulus (called a cue to action) is believed to be necessary to set the cognitive and behavioral processes in motion and is most clearly aligned with the therapeutic agent in the dosage metaphor. These cues can be either internal, such as symptoms, or external, such as a Public Service Announcement (PSA) on television or an interaction with friends or relatives.

The HBM includes communication explicitly as one of many potential cues to action that can influence behavior by modifying knowledge, attitudes, beliefs, group norms, and readiness to engage in the target behavior. Other variables such as demographic, sociopsychological, and structural variables are believed to indirectly impact on the outcome variable by their influence on individuals' threat perceptions and perceptions of the benefits of preventive actions (Rosenstock, 1990).

The HBM is still incomplete (Mikhail, 1981), with even its formulators adding variables from time to time, such as locus of control and self-efficacy (Rosenstock, Strecher, & Becker, 1988) and, most notably, a variable called health motivation (Becker et al., 1977). Health motivation refers to the degree of concern about health matters in general. This general health concern, which has been added as a third main component in the HBM, is believed to provide the motivation to make health issues salient and/or relevant. Saliency of health matters is believed to directly impact people's likelihood of taking some preventive health action (Rosenstock, Strecher, & Becker, 1988). In most empirical investigations the focus has been on the impact of the perceived threat and cost/benefit analysis of preventive health behaviors. Variables such as health motivation, (health) locus of control, self-efficacy, and cues to action have received almost no attention in empirical tests of the HBM (Rosenstock, 1990).

Similar to classic mass media approaches, the traditional HBM assigns a more passive role to individuals (Leventhal, Safer, & Panagis, 1983). However, individuals are likely to engage in health behaviors for proactive/wellness reasons as well as for threat-related ones (Leventhal, Safer, & Panagis, 1983). In addition, empirical tests of the HBM, while suggesting that its major variables have an impact on these processes, also suggest that there are other factors, not currently specified in the model, which may have pronounced effects (Calnan, 1984; Rosenstock, Strecher, & Becker, 1988). In general, the thrust of the model is on individually based psychosocial factors (Janz & Becker, 1984), not on the broader social context, including the information environment, in which individuals are embedded. This social context plays a critical role in an individual's self-regulation (Leventhal, Safer, & Panagis, 1983).

The major weakness of the HBM for our purposes is its very limited treatment of communication variables and its lack of attention to characteristics of the source of the message and the manner in which a message is presented, although later discussions of the model suggested that factors related to number and type of source should be incorporated in it (Rosenstock, Strecher, & Becker, 1988). Thus, as in many administrative approaches to campaigns, communication and the related need for persuasion are often taken for granted by health professionals (Becker & Rosenstock, 1984). Although not necessarily sanguine about its general benefit, the HBM's formulators do concede that in certain cases persuasive information can result in better adherence through the use of multiple channels and the reduction of complexity (Becker & Rosenstock, 1984). Interestingly, the model does not specifically include these issues since it does not go much beyond cues to action as a communication variable.

Transtheoretical Model

The Transtheoretical Model (TM) of behavior change introduced by Prochaska and DiClemente (1983, 1985, 1986) was developed from a systematic review of the psychotherapeutic literature in the context of smoking cessation. This model focuses on intentional change on the part of the individual and therefore has direct implications for how receptive people might be to change as the result of a dose of particular therapeutic agents (Prochaska, DiClemente, & Norcross, 1992). There is considerable evidence that this model can be applied to a wide range of health problems (Prochaska & DiClemente, 1985; Prochaska, DiClemente, & Norcross, 1992). Originally it suggested there were five basic processes of change: (1) consciousness raising, (2) catharsis, (3) commitment, (4) conditional stimuli, and (5) contingency management. These original processes have been modified and elaborated in subsequent research to as many as 13 separate processes of intentional change (DiClemente & Prochaska, 1985).

Difficulties in coping can result from three different problems with these processes (DiClemente & Prochaska, 1985). First, individual ignorance of these processes could result in a restricted range of responses. Second, an individual could be inept in implementing one of these processes. Third, an individual might prematurely implement a later process without going through all the necessary steps. When an individual experiences stress related to a perceived medical problem, two general coping options are available: the problem solving or instrumental option involves a direct behavioral response, while the other option involves the self-regulation of emotional stress (DiClemente & Prochaska, 1985).

The TM suggests readiness to engage in the target behavior falls along a continuum with implied sequencing, beginning with precontemplation, contemplation, decision making, active change, and maintenance (DiClemente & Prochaska, 1985). Contemplators are seriously considering taking action and are most concerned with consciousness raising. Any information they gather also will interact with their individual beliefs of self-efficacy in determining the likelihood that they will take action (DiClemente & Prochaska, 1985). Communication at later stages is likely to be used to confirm and reinforce a decision that individuals have already made, to keep them from wavering and relapsing to their original behavior. Still, even relapsers, people who are smoking again, often desire information related to their next attempt to quit smoking, with the argument made that they are enhancing their perception of self-efficacy, which is critical to their decision to try again (DiClemente & Prochaska, 1985).

Health campaign messages can be targeted to specific phases of readiness (e.g., messages targeting individuals who are at the precontemplation phase). This should enhance the prospects for change, given the assumption that additional, well-conceived targeting is usually beneficial. Indeed, the inclusion of the different phases of readiness implies that legitimate secondary outcome measures (e.g., increasing the percentage of a defined population that moves from precontemplation to contemplation) exist for other than "behavior change." The ability to measure and examine changes along the full spectrum of readiness is viewed as critical to a complete understanding of the overall impact of campaigns within defined populations and is one reason behind the TM's popularity; it also has implications for sequencing in a dosage metaphor.

Sensation Seeking

The sensation seeking targeting (SENTAR) approach developed at the University of Kentucky relies fundamentally on the application of the dosage metaphor (Palmgreen et al., 2002). Originally this approach was developed for the context of adolescent drug usage, a setting where sensation seeking is particularly important. Since then it has been expanded and applied to a broader array of contexts. Fundamentally this approach rests on the assumption of match: those with higher needs for sensation will seek stronger sources of stimulation; those with lower needs will seek weaker sources. So low sensation seekers will reject stimuli that are highly intense, preferring the familiar and less complex (Donohew et al., 2003).

This approach rests on four principles: (1) sensation seeking levels should be used to segment audiences, (2) formative research should be conducted on audience members to determine their level of sensation seeking, (3) prevention messages should be designed to match these levels, and (4) campaign messages should be placed in the context of similarly high sensation seeking value programming. Drawing from an activation model of information exposure, the SENTAR approach suggests then that persuasion is best achieved by using messages that appeal to individuals' fundamental approaches to seeking stimulation (Donohew et al., 2003). Fundamentally, then, this approach argues that the level of sensation seeking is a critical factor in determining whether or not messages will reach a receptive audience; dose is then determined by where audience members stand along this continuum.

Research on SENTAR has employed very sophisticated designs, such as the 32-month controlled interrupted time series switching replication in Fayette County, Kentucky, and Knoxville, Tennessee, which was intimately tied to frequency and amount issues.[2] This research also uniquely employed paid advertisements and the services of a professional media buyer. The campaign achieved its objectives in terms of penetration of the target audience of high sensation seeking adolescents, as well as their frequency of exposure. The results indicated substantial effects on the target audience and an important drop of about 25% for the absolute level of their marijuana usage (Donohew et al., 2003). Contrary to conventional wisdom, this study also may indicate that in certain circumstances, a media campaign alone can have significant impacts on behaviors.

CAMPAIGNS

How best to combine nicotine replacement and feasible "doses" of behavioral advice and support in primary care settings remains a critical research problem (Lichtenstein & Glasgow, 1992, p. 522).

Somewhat akin to mass media's historical bullet theory, discussed in chapter 5, then, the public was initially thought to be a relatively passive, defenseless audience. Public communication campaigns represent "purposive attempts to inform, persuade, or motivate behavior changes in a relatively well-defined and large audience, generally for noncommercial benefits to the individuals and/or society, typically within a given time period, by means of organized communication activities involving the mass media and often complemented by interpersonal support" (Rice & Atkin, 1989, p. 7).

In part because of the growing availability of federal funds for health-related communication campaigns, the 1960s and 1970s saw a resurgence of interest in campaigns and a feeling that they can succeed in certain circumstances (Noar, 2006). (Box 7.1 details the Stanford campaigns from this era.) This

---

BOX 7.1. THE STANFORD CAMPAIGNS

Most notable during the early 1970s was the Stanford Three Community Study (TCS) and later the Five City Project (FCP) (Flora, Maccoby, & Farquhar, 1989; Rimal, Flora, & Schooler, 1999). These campaigns were designed to reduce the epidemic rise in cardiovascular disease that was linked to specific lifestyle behaviors. They purposively used community approaches to changing individuals through an eclectic approach to borrowing theory from a wide variety of sources, from macrolevel to individual behavior changes, later described as the Communication-Behavior Change model. This model started with media messages that gained attention and provided information, then proceeded to face-to-face communication for providing incentives and role models, and then to community events that provided training, cues to action, and support for self-management skills. Planning for the campaign was based on assessing the distance between the baseline of particular individual behaviors and specific outcome objectives, then matching optimal interventions based on these assessments. The TCS uses a quasi-experimental design of a randomly selected panel of participants, aged 35 to 59, in each of the three cities for each of three years. One of the cities served as a control, while the other two cities varied the application of mass media and interpersonal approaches. Generally the results demonstrated a stronger impact for the media plus interpersonal intervention than the media-only intervention and control community. While demonstrating, especially for knowledge gain, that the media alone could produce changes for certain behaviors, other behaviors such as smoking cessation required considerable use of interpersonal interventions.

The more ambitious FCP followed with enhancements in terms of both design, including more formative evaluation, and interventions in the late 1970s. More sophisticated approaches to channel analysis were used for determining the reach, number of persons exposed, and frequency, measured by

continued

BOX 7.1.   *Continued*

the number messages for each exposed person of the media using during the campaign. More careful segmentation of the audience was also done along such factors as obesity. This study much more carefully operationalized issues relating to dosage and could link to actual campaign effects: "Remembered message percentages showed how the specification of the 'dose' of the intervention can increase your understanding of the 'response' in campaign outcomes" (Flora, Maccoby & Farquhar, 1989, pp. 250).

resulted, interestingly, in blame for unsuccessful campaigns being shifted from the recipients of the messages to the designers of the campaigns (Noar, 2006).

In the contemporary *conditional effects era*, successful campaign principles embody the dosage metaphor: increase exposure, develop properly targeted messages, and deliver them frequently (Noar, 2006). It is now widely recognized that mass media alone are unlikely to have the desired impacts; they must be supplemented with interpersonal communication within social networks (Noar, 2006). Modern campaigns, then, analyze a range of potential delivery systems, assessing such features of them as access, reach, and credibility (Silk, Atkin, & Salmon, 2011).

Campaigns fail when their audience questions their recommended beneficial effects and they do not tailor their messages to the audience's specific needs (Robertson & Wortzel, 1977). Prepackaged campaigns fail to realize that some people are active information seekers who persuade themselves when they discover satisfactory answers in their quest to answer their own questions (Freimuth, Stein, & Kean, 1989). This suggests that finer-grain discriminations of the audience may be necessary to insure effective communication, much as in emerging approaches to personalized medicine.

The tailoring of messages detailed in box 7.2 seeks to achieve a "match" between the information carriers health professionals choose to disseminate information and the desired outcomes of seekers (Dijkstra, Buijtels, & VanRaaij, 2005). Thus, the question becomes the much more sophisticated one of placing the most appropriate content in the most appropriate channel, where it is most likely to be used by a predetermined audience. This also results in much more efficient use of campaign resources (Silk, Atkin, & Salmon, 2011).

Health professionals' efforts also suffer from unrealistic expectations (Atkin, 1979). Most advertising campaigns would be happy with a level of change in their audience of 3% to 5% a year (Robertson & Wortzel, 1977). Typical of the expectations of health communicators, Cole and Wagner

---

BOX 7.2.   TAILORING

Tailoring approaches wed traditional campaign messages with very sophisticated segmenting technologies to more effectively reach audiences. They take on some of the characteristics of personalized medicine approaches with greater knowledge of individual characteristics, resulting in very specific strategies for influencing them. Contemporary approaches to tailoring offer the promise of systematically measuring dosage amounts and proper sequencing of messages (Morgan, King, & Ivic, 2011). They have become very popular approaches with over 500 research studies (Lustria et al., 2009) aimed at such behaviors as smoking, binge drinking, and diet. Most tailoring is based on demographic characteristics, but some has been done based on information needs, stages of change, and risk factors (Noar, Banac, & Harris, 2007). Media usage, a way of capturing delivery systems in the dosage metaphor, has also been suggested as a useful way of segmenting audiences for tailored messages (Rodgers et al., 2007).

More sophisticated tailoring approaches mimic some classic attributes of interpersonal channels on issues like changing messages as a result of feedback and more carefully targeted persuasion messages aimed at overcoming resistance (Kukafka, 2005). The explosion of m-health applications also promotes intraindividual tailoring and the possibility of very dynamic, longitudinal interventions involving ipsative feedback that are focused on issues like exercise and weight loss (Riley et al., 2011). Message tailoring goes hand in hand with audience segmentation and has seen considerable advances over the last couple of decades, especially with the advent of new media and technologies that facilitate its application. There is evidence across a number of domains that tailoring is superior to nontailoring of messages for campaigns (Rimal & Adkins, 2003). This is in part based on the classic public health formulation that impact equals efficacy times reach, with tailoring argued to have both high efficacy and high reach when it is used in Web-based applications.

(1990) expressed disappointment that only 37% of the colorectal screening tests they distributed during a screening program were returned for testing. Compared to most commercial campaigns this is an astonishing level of success. McGuire (1989) has also pointed out the very low probabilities of success of communication campaigns given the long string of steps that must be fulfilled (e.g., first get the audience's attention), each of which only has moderate probability of success. The use of campaigns is also contradindicated when pervasive product marketing (e.g., soft drink commercials), powerful social norms, and addictive behaviors (Wakefield, Loken, & Hornik, 2010) are present.

The general conclusion now is that health campaigns can exert moderate to powerful influence on cognitive outcomes (e.g., learning), less influence in changing attitudes, and even less influence on behaviors (Silk, Atkin, & Salmon, 2011). It is now recognized that the average health communication campaign changes the behavior of about 8% of the population (Noar, 2006), or stated in another way, the average media campaign effect represented by the mean of correlations in a meta-analysis was 0.09 (L. B. Snyder & Hamilton, 2002). The content focus of the mass media campaigns can also produce different impacts, with those focusing on tobacco having strong evidence for impact and those focusing on breast feeding only having weak evidence (Wakefield, Loken, & Hornik, 2010).

It has generally been found that direct interpersonal attempts at persuasion are more effective, but they are costly and have limited penetration. This sort of calculation has typically resulted in cost-conscious campaign administrators choosing the mass media for campaigns since, in the end, more people can be reached, resulting in a greater yield of changes in targeted behavior. So, an interpersonally driven strategy may have a 25% effectiveness rate but only reach 10,000 people because of budget concerns, resulting in a yield of 2,500. A comparably priced mass media campaign might reach 1 million people, with an effectiveness rate of 0.5%, but in the end it will double the yield to 5,000 people whose behavior is changed. Analyses of this sort are quite detailed and comprehensive in the commercial world but proprietary. As a result, a science of dosage appears to be a unique resource closely held by those who benefit from persuading others. This was particularly true in the 2012 presidential campaign, when President Barack Obama assembled a team that had a very scientific and rigorous approach to campaign principles.

Systematic comparisons of different delivery systems suggest that more sophisticated, expensive, and complicated approaches do not always result in better outcomes (Dijkstra, Buijtels, & VanRaaij, 2005; Lichtenstein & Glasgow, 1992). Organizational safety campaigns have found better outcomes by keeping messages simple; too many specific details, safety rules, and safety procedures can actually result in diminished impact (Real, 2008).

SOCIAL MARKETING

Campaigns are an integral component of social marketing approaches, but only one component. Marketing approaches go beyond words to actually provide products and services. This is often critical to promoting a sense of efficacy, a critical component, as we have seen, in determining proactive responses to health problems in target populations. Marketing approaches often provide incentives, making "good offers" to promote and reinforce change. So, antiobesity campaigns in schools may provide free or low-cost nutritious lunches. Thus, making someone's environment more favorable with timely provision of accessible services with favorable costs and/or benefits, providing clear competitive advantages to advocated behaviors, becomes critical to effective social marketing efforts.

These efforts often rest on the classic four *p*'s: product, price, place, and promotion. Product consists of the actual product (e.g., food consumption), the core product (e.g., weight control), and the augmented product (e.g., tasty alternatives). Price is a major stumbling block to antiobesity efforts since a healthy diet is often a more expensive one. This necessitates some sort of subsidy provided by the government or other source for these marketing efforts to be sustained for the long haul. Food deserts (e.g., urban areas that lack access to fresh produce) also exacerbate these problems, making creative solutions like mobile markets on buses, akin to traveling libraries, available to people in these neighborhoods. Finally, promotion often rests on the principles of campaigns we have just covered in depth.

Many observers would also suggest a fifth *p*, policy, also needs to be added to encourage the adoption of particular behaviors. So obesity campaigns might benefit from their interactive effects with various government regulations, ranging from the choices available in government-sponsored school meal programs to Mayor Michael Bloomberg's much publicized initiative to limit the size of sugary soft drinks.

RISK COMMUNICATION

Risk communication is one of the fastest-growing areas of health communication. It seems like every week we face either an environmental catastrophe or a new alert about food-borne illnesses. There is also a general perception that the probability of disasters and the hazards associated with them are increasing as a result of climate change. Many of these hazards have profound implications for health.

While risks can be generalized and last for long periods of time, thus potentially permitting a wide range of communication strategies, crises imply high salience and the demand for an immediate response, limiting the types of messages and modalities that can be used to transmit them. While generally crises are considered to be "surprises," they can often be anticipated, but because they are often considered to be unlikely, organizations often do not spend sufficient time preparing for them or scanning the environment for potential threats. Often the handling of crises can make or break organizations and/or politicians. This is another example of a situation where one message, one dose, can permanently alter the relationships between interactants (Fischoff, 1995). For organizations the fundamental question that needs to be answered is, What is the social contract between those who create risks and those who must bear them (Fischoff, 1995)? Here we will not cover the personal, individualized communication of risks that are often central to interpersonal relationships between health care providers and clients that we focused on in chapter 3 or the personally risky behavior that is often the focus of the communication campaigns we focused on earlier in this chapter.

One of the most interesting things about risks is the disconnect between perceptions of them and the actual dangers people might face. So, many people dread flying, when it is far safer than going to the corner grocery store in your car. Generally people see greater risks in voluntary (e.g., skiing) than involuntary (e.g., being exposed to carcinogens in everyday food) activities. There are also dread risks and unknown risks that provoke high degrees of uncertainty, which people seek to overcome through communication. The holy grail of risk communication is the development of messages that can reduce the gap between perceived risk and actual probabilistic risk (Turner, Skubisz, & Rimal, 2011). Since risk perceptions are often socially constructed and rely on communication in their development, organizations often spend considerable efforts in trying to influence their development.

Because of their broad reach mass media often become central to the responses to crises and shaping risk perceptions more generally, with agenda setting and media dependency theories particularly useful. So, the media can identify the most central elements of a crisis that need to be dealt with, and they may be the exclusive source of information until normalcy returns.

Through social amplification processes, like the bandwidth and echo problems in social networks we discussed in chapter 4, messages often take on a life of their own in social systems and can be difficult to control. Organizations must engage in environmental scanning that evaluates the reactions of key stakeholders to their messages, as well as emerging countermessages that might be developing. In a crisis rumor control and dealing with uncertainties require very sophisticated monitoring and response groups. In today's very fragmented, high-speed media environment, organizations are foolhardy to assume that just because they have sent out a press release they have effectively responded to a crisis.

Organizations often have compelling interests in ameliorating perceptions of risk and crisis. Unfortunately their affected publics also may be associated with already existing problems of environmental justice and health disparities that make resistance to messages increasingly likely.

Because of the immediate responses needed, proper crisis preparation and, perhaps even more importantly, prevention activities can mitigate their effects. In this connection, organizations also need to be transparent about communicating risks to their various affected publics, stakeholders, and communities. When the crisis is upon us is not the best time to build relationships, especially since dealing with a crisis often entails a fair amount of trust among interactants.

Metaphors may be very useful tools for communicating emerging risks (Turner, Skubisz, & Rimal, 2011) and placing them in their proper frame. Definitions of a situation often entail appropriate responses and are thus critical to responses to risk and crisis communication events (Mileti & Beck, 1975). So focusing on heroic first responder narratives may distract the public's attention from the factors that led to the need for their efforts in the first place.

Risks are often communicated by probabilities, so innumeracy becomes an issue (Turner, Skubisz, & Rimal, 2011). This often contributes to differences in lay and expert perceptions of particular issues (Wright, Sparks, & O'Hair, 2008). The fundamental question being addressed here is, How safe is safe enough? For many members of the public, no level of risk is safe (Fischoff, 1995), particularly when it affects their own health or that of their children.

Numeracy is the ability to reason with numbers and to apply mathematics to solve quantitative problems. Studies indicate that half of the adult American population may be unsure how to calculate percentages and unable to understand probability statements (Paulos, 1989) or even, for that matter, what a percentage means (Blumenthal, 2010). Quantitative literacy is key to the promotion of prevention measures since many health issues are expressed in terms of statistical probability—the likelihood of contracting an illness or of a treatment being effective. In communicating probabilities graphic, visualization approaches might be particularly helpful, especially when communicating primary and secondary impacts and counterintuitive meanings (Anderson & Walsch, 2013).

How a health outcome (or other information) is *framed*, something organizations are becoming increasingly skilled at, has important consequences for patient decision making. People are more likely to accept scenarios presented with positive framing (e.g., survival rates from a treatment) than negative ones (e.g., likelihood of death from the same treatment) (Kahneman, Slovic, & Tversky, 1982; Rifkin & Bouwer, 2007; L. M. Schwartz et al., 1997).

It is especially important that baseline risk data be given that allows people to understand medical outcomes (e.g., how many women out of 1,000 are likely to die from breast cancer over a 10-year period) (L. M. Schwartz et al., 1997). Without baseline information, patients are more likely to have inaccurate perceptions of probabilities; for example, they can only imagine what a "33% reduction in risk" means, not truly understand the final probabilities (Malenka et al., 1993). However, expressions of relative risks are more likely to lead to perceptions of efficacy among patients, presumably due to the use of large percentages (e.g., 33%) rather than absolute numbers (e.g., 4 in 1,000).

When the social contract between an organization and the public is broken often, there is an underlying emotional response that must be dealt with. Successful anger, and even outrage, management often plays a significant role in the aftermath of a crisis. People often exhibit dysfunctional reactions to risks when they feel they have low efficacy (Rimal, 2001). So they may exhibit increased levels of anxiety and even indifference and avoidance when they feel there is nothing they can do. Information about possible threats creates tensions in the minds of audience members, who must in turn find some way to resolve it. If the threat is extreme, such as in some fear appeals often used in campaigns (see box 7.3), or if any potential responses are not expected to be effective, then an attractive alternative is to ignore the threat entirely—which in turn promotes consistency (Case et al., 2005).

BOX 7.3.   FEAR APPEALS

Fear appeals, such as those embedded in often gruesome but colorful warnings about cigarette smoking, seem to be inherently appealing to health communicators. However, the research evidence concerning their effectiveness is equivocal at best, and they present possible ethical problems for health communicators since they often heighten emotional arousal and exaggerate risks (Guttman, 2011). They also may be one of the classic cases of matching (Averbeck, Jones, & Robertson, 2011), with too much fear arousal leading to boomerang effects, especially among more resistant, marginalized populations, and too little fear arousal, not stimulating people to act. They also, as is the case for many other health communication messages, appear to work best when they are also coupled with messages concerning self-efficacy, that there is something the receiver can readily do in response to the message.

Research on "fear appeals" has emphasized another possibility: purposeful *rejection* of information. For example, Janis and Feshback (1953) found that extreme attempts to frighten people into practicing good dental hygiene—by showing them pictures of mouth cancer and deformed teeth—were not very effective. They hypothesized that such strong arousals led those exposed to "ignore" the threat, whereas milder portrayals were better at leading them to confront the underlying problem. Other researchers of fear appeals (e.g., Dillard, 1994; Witte, 1994) have teased out distinctions in the way that people evaluate information directed at them in mass media campaigns. Our attempts to control danger operate in parallel with the way we manage our fears and anxiety; we may protect ourselves from danger by accepting suggestions for avoiding the stimuli that provoke fear.

SUMMARY

Finally, accept that evaluations of public health communication programs will rarely produce the unequivocal evidence promised in randomized controlled trials of pills. Sometimes this is feasible for smaller scale trials, where enough resources can be mustered to produce a substantial additional dose of exposure . . . but most often this is not the case (Hornik, 2002b, p. 16).

A controlled clinical trial may make sense if the things to be studied is a discrete thing (a pill) that can be delivered or not delivered (Hornik, 2002b, p. 12).

Hornik (2002b) goes on to suggest, in a classic communication researcher's rebuttal of the dosage metaphor, that the diffusion of public communication messages is much messier, involving multiple messages from a variety of sources and widespread institutional and societal changes, reflecting emerging social trends. Of course, this also reveals a relatively primitive understanding of the dosage metaphor. Often today's treatments, for example for high blood pressure, involve multiple medications, behavioral changes, and changes in the patient's social milieu. Obviously the nature of the therapeutic agent, in this case most commonly messages, has a profound impact on the success of campaigns, as the SENTAR approach demonstrates.

A key difference found in a meta-analysis was that between campaigns that stress legal enforcement, coercion issues, and classic persuasion attempts (L. B. Snyder & Hamilton, 2002). Often campaigns fail because they neglect such basic elements of the dosage metaphor as ensuring widespread, frequent, and prolonged exposure to messages, and they tend not to focus on audience segmentation, a version of personalized medicine, or targeting (Palmgreen et al., 2002). Some have also explicitly noted a clear dose-response relationship to public health campaigns (Buller et al., 2008).

As table 7.1 suggests, earlier approaches to campaigns did not focus in a detailed or sophisticated way on amount and frequency elements of the dosage metaphor. How long a campaign should last to achieve effects is also a great unknown, as is the point at which a message reaches diminishing returns in terms of its repetition (Salmon & Atkin, 2003). More recent approaches to campaigns, interestingly involving communication researchers in their development, represented by sensation seeking approaches to campaigns, do specifically incorporate issues of amount and frequency. L. B. Snyder and M. A. Hamilton (2002) found evidence confirming that campaigns with greater reach, that is, a higher percentage of people exposed to campaign messages, having greater impacts, comparable to the importance of vaccination reaching a critical mass of the population. A major focus of some public communication campaigns is also to encourage people to seek other channels

Table 7.1. Comparing Behavioral Science Approaches and the Dosage Metaphor

| | *Behavioral Science Approach* | | |
Dosage Elements	*Health Belief Model*	*Transtheoretical Model*	*Sensation Seeking*
Amount	Not specified	Depends on staging	Increased exposure, dose/response
Frequency	One-shot	Depends on staging	Sophisticated designs
Sequencing	Cue to action	Progression through stages	Sophisticated designs
Delivery systems	Various	Not specified	Match stimulus
Interactions	Social norms, beliefs, social structure	Motivation, readiness, self-efficacy	Embedded in stimulus
Contraindications	Complexity, "intelligent noncompliance"	Wrong stage	Poor match, audience segmentation
Dysfunctions	Passivity, administrative science	Wasted effort, resistance	Wasted effort, resistance

for information, achieving both variety and delivery systems and repetition of messages (Salmon & Atkin, 2003).[3] A critical issue in determining the success of campaigns is insuring enough exposure for effects to be achieved (Stephenson, Southwell, & Yzer, 2011).

Campaign approaches do focus on an essential element of sequencing, or that one thing must follow another, although theoretical approaches are often inadequate to explain emerging m-health applications that are more interactive and adaptive to feedback (Riley et al., 2011). So cues to action are followed by appropriate mental processing, which then leads to health behaviors, and stages of change go through a predictable progression. The sensation seeking approach comes close to predicting the rate of change in longitudinal approaches based on the exposure of people to messages over time. Another critical issue in the evaluation of health communication campaigns is the expected lag before the campaign is likely to have an impact (Hornik, 2002a). For example, looking at the last three decades, there have been dramatic drops in smoking. However, if we change the evaluation to a yearly one, drops are only in the 1% to 2% range.

Unfortunately, there isn't the same sophistication in terms of a range of delivery systems, in part because of the traditional mass media focus of campaigns, but this is changing in response to the proliferation of new media. Although the Stanford studies used a variety of channels, including, classically, interpersonal ones for persuasion, the sensation seeking approach offers interesting arguments in terms of the content of the campaign related to high sensation seeking, suggesting messages need to be embedded in media that is favored by high sensation seekers, somewhat evocative of Marshall McLuhan's famous observation that the medium is the message.

A general problem with mass media communication campaign evaluation is that often intervention efforts stem from widespread recognition that change is needed, resulting in a population moving in the desired direction of any one campaign (Fan, 2002). As a result, campaign effects, if any, are contaminated by uncontrolled messages, interacting with those found in the mass media generally. The ever-present risk of contamination by secular trends highlights the importance of control groups in research designed to evaluate campaign impacts (L. B. Snyder & Hamilton, 2002).

Often contraindications focus on issues of match. So willingness to change, the wrong stage, poor audience segmentation, and lack of understanding of social network differentiation can all lead to failed campaigns.

Beyond the wasted resources of poorly designed campaigns there has been little consideration of dysfunctional aspects of campaign approaches, perhaps because of their implicit roots in administrative science and a general feeling that those in authority know what's best. A great unknown, relating to campaign sequencing effects, is their decay rate (L. B. Snyder & Hamilton, 2002), which is also a classic issue related to dosage impacts, with parallels to the flushing of drugs from the system, and a very important consideration when a behavior that is advocated by a campaign (e.g., breast self-exams) later turns out to be not as efficacious as first thought. As in any paternalistic approach, there are general problems with campaign's and risk communication's top-down approach, resulting in passive or dependent reactive audiences who do not engage in "intelligent noncompliance."

NOTES

1. Totalitarian campaigns, with the Maoists in Communist China perhaps the most sophisticated, also have been developed using similar principles. They will not be our focus here.

2. Often, when immediate results are not seen for a public campaign, the argument is made that there was not a cumulative effect due to a prolonged repetition of the message or an adequate dosage.

3. In an interesting twist, the individual thus serves as the agent of his or her own targeting.

FURTHER READINGS

Noar, S. M. (2005–2006). A health educator's guide to theories of health behavior. *International Quarterly of Community Health Education, 24* (1), 75–92.
Review of the numerous theories that form a basis for health interventions written for health professionals; provides guidelines for choosing a theory, then applying it to particular problems.

Noar, S. M. (2006). A 10-year retrospective of research in health mass media campaigns: Where do we go from here? *Journal of Health Communication, 11,* 21–42. doi: 10.1080/10810730500461059.
Comprehensive review of factors leading to effective campaigns with exemplars of campaigns that followed particular strategies (e.g., audience segmentation). This article also suggests future areas for research on mass media campaigns.

Turner, M. M., Skubisz, C., & Rimal, R. N. (2011). Theory and practice in risk communication: A review of the literature and visions of the future. In T. L. Thompson, R. Parrott, & J. F. Nussbaum (Eds.), *The Routledge handbook of health communication* (2nd ed., pp. 146–164). New York: Routledge.
Comprehensive review of communication approaches to risk, an increasingly important area of health communication research; published in the most comprehensive resource for health communicators.

Health Information Technology

> Cutting-edge technology, especially in communication and information transfer, will enable the greatest advances yet in public health. Real health care reform will come only from demand reduction, as individuals learn to take charge of their health. . . . Communication technology can work wonders for us in this vital endeavor . . . encouraging personal wellness and prevention and leading to better informed decisions about health care (Koop, 1995, p. 760).

*H*ealth information technology (HIT) has recently been the subject of substantial investments, in part because it is often seen as a solution to our inordinately costly and often inefficient health care system (Riley et al., 2011; T. G. Thompson & Brailer, 2004). A number of metaphors have frequently been used to describe the impacts of information technologies, including lever, web, machine in the garden, and revolution. So new technologies are levers that extend human capabilities and, as in a physical garden, provide an environment in which individuals can thrive (Kaplan, 1990). The web itself has been suggested to be best understood by the metaphor of managerial rhetoric (Kent, 2001). Some new features of the Internet, such as portals, which in turn often rely on the application of metaphors for enhanced understanding, like gateways, billboards, networks, niches, and brands, rest on metaphors (Kalyanaraman & Sundar, 2008).

Technology, of course, has many benefits. First, it increases access both in terms of electronic propinquity, bringing people closer together, and in terms of scale, with worldwide access to sources that are often intercultural or international (Pfister & Soliz, 2011). Second, it provides an ever-increasing array of tools (e.g., delivery systems) for on-demand, real-time inquiry into pressing questions that people may have. These tools often have a wide range of properties (e.g., interactivity) and can activate many senses, increasing their social presence and resulting engagement. Third, technology provides unique context spaces for interactions (e.g., chat rooms) that often blend dialogue and dissemination (Pfister & Soliz, 2011). Fourth, because of the increasing flood of information available multiple means of delegation/gatekeeping have emerged that encourage disintermediation and the breakup of the monopoly that the professions once held on health information. So, although health information technology is creating a flood of information that people are increasingly having difficulty controlling, it is also creating new opportunities for self-administration and controlling doses. Fifth, this has also led to the increasing importance of the self-administration of doses of information, with individuals deciding for themselves how much to acquire and how frequently.

As a result of these enhanced capabilities, increasingly health professionals are turning to technology to facilitate their work. While they are traditionally slow to adopt new media, e-health and, more recently, m-health apps are changing the world of health communicators. However, in spite of often rosy predictions, the impact of information-processing technologies has been a matter of some controversy, as has their relationship to productivity, profitability, quality, and competitive advantage. In the health arena a variety of contextual factors have limited the application of technologies: doctors' traditional resistance; expense; changing relationships among the professions; a federal system that has created a welter of regulations, privacy laws, and so on; and competing hospital, insurance, and vendor systems (J. D. Johnson, 2009c).

At a fundamental level, technology may be defined simply as actions employed to transfer inputs into outputs. It can be viewed not just in the narrow sense of focusing on machines needed to produce physical goods but in the broader sense of any systematic set of techniques. In this chapter we will explore in more detail how HITs are promoting access, facilitating information seeking, increasing engagement, enhancing decision making, and providing means for controlling access to an overwhelming flood of information that threatens to overdose all of us.

PROMOTING ACCESS

One of the most exciting contemporary movements relating to technology is its facilitation of social contacts, which promote collaboration, the sharing of information, and the development of communities. More than half of online health information seekers do so for someone else and discuss such information with others (Fox & Jones, 2009). Online support groups foster patient empowerment or management (Barak, Boniel-Nissim, & Suler, 2008), and participation tools may lead to more positive outcomes, especially for rare diseases (Wicks et al., 2010).

The Internet may be the ultimate game changer for health communicators. It has made possible access to an often bewildering array of authoritative (and nonauthoritative) information, allowing people to self-administer dosages. Broadly speaking, Eysenbach (2005) has identified four levels of accessibility: physical, findability, readability and comprehendability, and usability. The Internet has ameliorated some of the problems with physical access and certainly has promoted vastly improved tools for finding information. However, the last two dimensions of accessibility present some real challenges for health communicators, given very grave limitations in health literacy and access to health care once a problem is identified.

This is coupled with a growing interest among our federal agencies in health disparities. In general, it has been argued that there is a growing difference in access to information between different segments of our society and that, increasingly, this gap also reflects other demographic classifications, such as socioeconomic status, leading to the focus on the knowledge gap and information poor we discussed in chapter 5.

Another major impediment for health communication relating to some groups is a lack of necessary information-processing skills, some as fundamental as literacy and knowledge of the primary language in which most health matters are expressed (Freimuth, Stein, & Kean, 1989). The information fields in which the poor are embedded typically involve one-way communication from mass entertainment-oriented media, such as television (Freimuth, Stein, & Kean, 1989). Added to this mix of impediments is a possibility of mistrust and deliberate rejection of what is seen as "establishment" positions (Freimuth, Stein, & Kean, 1989). Health communication clearly differs by educational level. So, not only is it important to provide access to the Internet (see box 8.1), but people also must receive the training necessary to use it (J. D. Johnson & Case, 2012). In addition, technology and software access is likely to be greater for privileged groups within our society, contributing to the knowledge gap discussed in chapter 5.

New technologies and new media also create an increasingly fragmented and privatized information environment, as opposed to the more mass, public access technologies represented by television and radio. As we saw in box 5.2, health professionals in important ways have lost control of the message, and they can't set the agenda of what the public will attend to since their exclusive control over information resources is steadily declining, raising concerns about self-administration of medical doses. "Bad ideas spread more rapidly among the ignorant than among the informed, and good ideas spread more rapidly among the informed than the ignorant" (March, 1994, p. 246).

BOX 8.1. INTERNET SEARCHING

Health information is ubiquitous on the Internet. It is usually described as the second- or third-most likely reason people go to Internet sites. There is no shortage of sites focused on a variety of issues, ranging from selling products to psychosocial adjustment to omnibus sites that cover a range of different contents. So someone who wants to self-administer a dose of information literally has no limit on issues like amount, frequency, sequencing, and range of delivery systems.

Of course, there is a darker side to the Internet, with sites that are untrustworthy for a variety of reasons (e.g., underlying commercial motivations, outdatedness, reliance on quackery, and on and on). The Internet also can exacerbate underlying societal inequalities and access to health care, in part because the information it contains is often overwhelming in its volume and detail, contributing to information overload (Cotten & Gupta, 2004). Most Internet users want "just-in-time" information and are impressed with surface characteristics of sites (e.g., visual attractiveness) (Eysenbach, 2005), and they do not exhibit much concern with such issues as trustworthiness and quality.

Whom do you trust? The Internet, of course, is unregulated, which is one of its charms, but this also means that users must be constantly vigilant concerning commercial motivations and hidden agendas. Many sites are essentially advertorials or glorified press releases with exaggerated claims. An interesting site that tries to monitor some of the worst abuses relating to health is Quackwatch (http://www.quackwatch.com).

There are also real questions concerning the quality of information on many sites, which is especially troublesome since most people don't systematically evaluate the quality of information they get on the Web (Crespo, 2004). There are many ways to evaluate the quality of sites. Do they provide peer-reviewed information that multiple experts have vetted? Is the information evidence based? Have there been timely updates of information? Is it comprehensive? Does it present two sides? Does it suggest you should consult your physician or provide other sources of information? Does it have an "about us" page that details its editorial/review policy, privacy protections, and contact information? Does the site display an HONcode of principles, which in effect is a "Good Housekeeping Seal of Approval" (Crespo, 2004)?

Of course, there are other factors that contribute to the usefulness of a particular site. One of the most important of these is, Does it promote interactivity and user engagement? For example, does it feature human-to-human interaction either with a professional, like Cancer Information Services Live Help, or with other people who are dealing with a particular illness?

There is a whole host of other qualities that also contribute to a user's evaluation of a site. Is it easy to navigate? What is its intended audience in terms of issues like level of health literacy and numeracy required to interpret information on the site. (The Medical Library Association has a helpful cite for deciphering health information: http://mlanet.org/resources/medspeak/medspeak.html.)

One of the best general sites for health information is Medline Plus (http://www.nlm.nih.gov/medlineplus), which is a service of the National Library of Medicine of the National Institutes of Health. It has over 20,000 links to informational and printable webpages. It is sensitive to issues of health literacy and has information in nearly 50 languages. It has very creative visuals and interactive tutorials, including videos of actual surgical procedures. Its medical encyclopedia is updated quarterly. It also allows users to sign up for e-mail announcements that keep them up to date on new developments. It has interactive features like games, calculators, and quizzes. Its descriptions of diseases describe symptoms, causes, exams and tests, treatment, outlook, possible complications, when to contact a medical professional, and prevention. This site, then, is sensitive to the need for multiple delivery systems that can, in effect, enhance the dosage of any information obtained.

FACILITATING

Creating rich information fields through such practices as "self-serving" to information from databases should make for more informed consumers who will likely take up less of health professionals' time "being brought up to speed" on the basics of their disease and its treatment, since they can self-administer. Developing a wide range of delivery systems from which to choose to administer a dose and facilitating access to them has become a popular strategy for encouraging people to regulate their own doses of information. This is especially so for the new technologies associated with personal information management detailed in box 8.2.

Knowledge management (KM) has been loosely applied to a collection of practices related to generating, capturing, storing, disseminating, and applying knowledge (Stewart, 2001). More effective KM should lead to better decision making and a flourishing of creative approaches to problems. In the United States, governments have made substantial investments in information infrastructure, in part to encourage the more rapid dissemination of information (Hesse, Johnson, & Davis, 2010). The US National Institutes of Health, primarily through the National Library of Medicine, in particular has devoted considerable resources and thought to building a national information infrastructure related to health. This has been done partially to respond to the concerns of advocacy groups for

BOX 8.2.   PERSONAL INFORMATION MANAGEMENT

Personal information management is a form of intrapersonal communication that may prevent unnecessary repetition of doses. Keeping good searchable records can be critical to health care. Some models of information seeking suggest that the first step in a search process is that someone evaluates his or her current information (Freimuth, Stein & Kean 1989), a task that is made much easier if one has kept careful records.

As Katrina demonstrated, paper records stored in the offices of medical providers may lead to substantial problems when those records are either unavailable for long periods or destroyed. The advent of electronic medical records can address some of these problems, but there are many competing systems, and it is often difficult to share records across them for both technical and institutional reasons.

One of the most exciting developments today comes in the area of m-health, which combines mobile applications with sensors. So, RunKeeper employs a phone's GPS to track running and cycling and, through its Health Graph feature, allows users to track their performance. The Boozerlyzer measures blood alcohol levels, and Green Goose's sticker-size sensors can transmit data on usage of everyday objects like toothbrushes (Mongalindan, 2012). These tools address some of the barriers to adoption that have hindered the adoption of personal information management systems in the past.

Manually entered data or data from sensors can then be entered into personal information management software systems that also can provide decision support and are often very useful in managing chronic diseases. However, manual entry of data is often cumbersome and raises questions of accuracy. These issues are being addressed by an explosion of sensor-based applications that make data collection nearly automatic. There are also movements to make these systems compatible with downloads of records from physician's offices. Downloading doctor's notes also creates the possibility of the patient correcting errors.

However, there are a number of problems with these systems, not the least of which is that individuals have been slow to adopt them. There are also substantial concerns with privacy since the underlying business model is often based on selling aggregated health information to drug companies and others. There are also potential problems with obsessive behavior, overdoses if you will. So some commentators have described early adopters of these systems as "quant junkies" (Mongalindan, 2012) or "trackers" who are obsessed with quantifying themselves and increasingly treat their bodies as a project. It has been recently found that some 70% of Americans keep track of personal health information (e.g., blood pressure, glucose levels), but they do so mostly informally, in their heads. Nearly half of these trackers say that this self-monitoring has helped them manage their own health or that of a person they care for (Paddock, 2013). This continuing sequencing of doses then becomes very important for people coping with chronic health problems.

more rapid dissemination of knowledge, particularly related to AIDS and breast cancer. Rather than stressing simple access to ideas, it may be better to stress access to playful intellectual tools that allow individuals to make sense of an overwhelming information environment (Entman & Wildman, 1992). Accordingly, agencies have increasingly encouraged creative approaches to information dissemination, including gaming, which we will discuss in more detail in a later section.

There also has been increasing use of secondary information disseminators, or brokers, which is really a variant on classic notions of opinion leadership (Katz, 1957; Katz & Lazersfeld, 1955) and gatekeepers (Metoyer-Duran, 1993). Opinion leadership suggests ideas flow from the media to opinion leaders to those *less active* segments of the population. Opinion leaders not only serve a relay function, however, but also provide social support information to individuals, reinforce messages by their social influence over them, and validate the authoritativeness of the information (Paisley, 1994). So, not only do opinion leaders serve to disseminate ideas, but they also, because of the interpersonal nature of their ties, provide additional pressure to conform as well. Another trend in this area is the recognition of human gatekeepers, community-based individuals who can provide information to at-risk individuals (Metoyer-Duran, 1993) and refer them to more authoritative sources for treatments (J. D. Johnson & Meischke, 1993a, 1993b). Recognizing the powers of peer opinion leaders, many health institutions are establishing patient advocacy programs. So, cancer survivors can serve to guide new patients through their treatments.

Gatekeeping in its various forms is seen as a key differentiating feature of the Internet, consisting of collective gatekeeping (e.g., bulletin boards, wikis), individual gatekeeping (e.g., blogs, social networking sites), and unknown gatekeeping (Sundar et al., 2011). The possibilities for gatekeeping proliferate every day. Brokers overcome the incompleteness of these institutional designs to achieve various types of information technology integration. Knowledge brokers address the following problems: converting tacit to explicit knowledge, addressing individual cynicism and resistance to change, overcoming cultural barriers, developing familiarity with professional norms, and recognizing broader trends.

J. D. Johnson (2004) identified four key sets of variables critical to the effectiveness of brokers that have traditionally been identified in the literature: homophily, trust, shared interests/threats, and differentiation/integration. His approach stresses the balance between shared interests and threats that emerge in relationships with other groups. It also links these factors to homophily, a key feature of modern demographic theory (Monge & Contractor, 2003), as well as a continuing foundational factor in communication theory (Rogers, 2003). Central to both systems theory and structuralist explanations of problems that develop in intergroup relationships is the balance between differentiation and integration (J. D. Johnson, 1993a). Finally, market-driven approaches stress that trust is the most important factor in knowledge brokering and managing risks (Dai & Kauffman, 2002; Davenport & Prusak, 1998), with the national information infrastructure both increasing ways of monitoring trust and diminishing the needs for interpersonal contact that have been its traditional basis.

There are a number of ways that the use of third parties, particularly knowledge brokers, can complement clinical practice. First, individuals who want to be fully prepared before they visit the doctor often consult the Internet. In fact, Lowery and Anderson (2002) suggest that prior information use may impact respondents' perception of physicians. However, physicians often have difficulty with conversations with patients concerning information gathered on the Internet (Sabee et al., 2012). Second, there appears to be an interesting split among Internet users, with as many as 60% of users reporting that while they look for information, they only rely on it if their doctors tell them to (H. Taylor & Leitman, 2002). While the Internet makes a wealth of information available for particular purposes, it is often difficult for the novitiate to weigh the credibility of the information, a critical service that a knowledge broker, such as a clinical professional or consumer health librarian, can provide. This suggests that a precursor to a better patient-doctor dialogue would be to increase the public's knowledge base and to provide alternative but complementary information sources by shaping clients' information fields. Flay and his colleagues (Flay, 1987; Flay, DiTecco, & Schlegel, 1980) have found that to induce behavioral change regarding health promotion, a message must be repeated over a long period via multiple sources, thereby increasing the dose. By shaping and influencing the external sources a patient will consult both before and after visits, clinical practices can, at one and the same time, reduce their own burden of explaining (or defending) their approach and increase the likelihood of patient compliance. While it is well known that individuals often consult a variety of others before presenting themselves in clinical settings (J. D. Johnson, 1997a), outside HMO and organization contexts, there have been few systematic attempts to shape the nature of these prior consultations. If these prior information searches happen in a relatively uncontrolled, random, parallel manner, expectations (e.g., treatment options, diagnosis, drug regimens) may be established that will be unfulfilled in the clinical encounter.

The emergence of the Internet as an omnibus source of information has apparently changed the nature of opinion leadership; both more authoritative (e.g., medical journals and literature) and more interpersonal (e.g., support or advocacy groups) sources are readily available and accessible online. This is part of a broader trend that A. L. Shapiro (1999) refers to as "disintermediation," or the capability of the Internet to allow the general public to bypass experts in the quest for information, products, and services. The risk here, however, is that individuals can quickly become overloaded or confused in an undirected environment. In essence, while the goal may be to reduce uncertainty or help bridge a knowledge gap, the actual effect can be increased uncertainty and, ultimately, decreased sense of efficacy for future searches. A focus on promoting health information literacy, then, would mean helping people gain the skills to access, judge the credibility of, and effectively utilize a wide range of health information. Though intermediaries play an important role despite more consumer health information on the Internet, increasing health literacy by encouraging autonomous information seeking also should be a goal of our health care system.

Self-Help Groups

Increasingly, more formal groups are serving as opinion leaders and information seekers for, or supporting the information needs of, individuals. Self-help groups are estimated to be in the hundreds of thousands across a wide variety of diseases, with members numbering in the millions (Barak, Boniel-Nissim, & Suler, 2008). They also can provide critical information on the personal side of disease: How will my spouse react? Am I in danger of losing my job? Will I get proper treatment in a clinical study?

Driving this movement has been the notion that self-help groups have the potential to affect outcomes by supporting patients' general well-being and sense of personal empowerment (Barak, Boniel-Nissim, & Suler, 2008), and the diverse tools now available have the potential to further enable this. Enhanced access to others willing to share experiences is obviously critical and certainly was much more difficult prior to the information and communication technologies available today that facilitate the sort of social networking discussed in box 8.3.

The notion of the "expert patient" has gained increased attention, particularly in rare diseases, given the amount and variety of information available on the Internet, the concern by some health professionals that patients may challenge existing power structures (though many others encourage knowledge acquisition by patients), and the increased ability to form communities (Ayme, Kole, & Groft, 2008).

There continues to be a shift from traditional models of medicine and medical research to one where patients have a greater role in their own decisions, from treatment options, to involvement in clinical research, to actually initiating and driving research. More than to simple choice, the core issues relate to choice for the purpose of more personalized care, to increase safety in research and care, and for other altruistic purposes that require social networks that can enable knowledge transfer, greater voice, and concerted action.

BOX 8.3.   SOCIAL MEDIA AND SOCIAL NETWORKING

Social media services are primarily technology and software facilitators for people to form relationships with each other. Typically, they define a universe of users, entities, through directories. They also can define the types of relationships users would like to have with others. Users are often seen to be members of particular communities, and in some applications social networking sites facilitate the development of crowd sourcing around particular interests and activities.

Recent examples of social media applied to health problems are many: online games where teams try to identify causes; tweeting simple symptoms to a user community, asking for input; posting symptoms on blogs, websites, asking for feedback; and posting photos of dermatological features on Facebook, asking for comment (Park, 2012).

The content features of these websites, especially in terms of facilitating the flow of complex information in various forms (e.g., graphic, visual, and so on), form one of the reasons for the excitement underlying their application to health. These features have been associated with the development of Web 2.0, which encourages the development of collective intelligence through the participation of users (Boulos & Wheeler, 2007).

Technologies associated with the sites enhance a number of differing possibilities for interacting, delivery systems if you will: babble, chat, blasts, blogging, discussion boards, e-mail, loops, pokes, requests, reviews, shouts, tagging, trackback ping, and so on.

Reciprocity is not individually based but communal. For dyadic reciprocity access to more detailed information is often dependent on both parties agreeing that they have a relationship of a particular sort (e.g., friendship). However, in the social media world, often more altruistic, community-based motivations appear to be present. People gain standing in the community through their input; they also often have a common collective goal they want to advance, such as improved treatment for chronic diseases. To achieve maximum benefits, like in other communication technologies, critical mass obviously makes a big difference.

These sites increasingly provide unique sources of information. They enhance the potential, then, to identify weak ties that may have critical information. So Myspace's browse function allowed searches through extended networks for people meeting particular demographic classifications, and its search feature allowed you to try to find people by affiliations. Social network sites can make visible more indirect contacts (e.g., friends of friends), thus facilitating the development of other ties.

Social media sites offer considerable possibilities for sharing and transferring information that can also enhance creativity and innovation. So one can transcend physical, cultural, and social boundaries to get access to needed information. In Ev Rogers's terms, they can turbocharge someone's existing network. They facilitate the development of communities of practice around particular interests and activities, such as Yahoo! groups. These sites often move beyond just sharing advice to encouraging activism and the aggregation of data from users that can approach classic scientific approaches to research on diseases.

Increasingly more formal groups are serving as opinion leaders and information seekers for individuals. A big advantage of patient-centered support groups is speed, since waiting for scientific certainty can be lethal (Ferguson, 2007). They also can provide critical information on the personal side of disease: How will my children react? Can I continue schooling? And so on.

INCREASING ENGAGEMENT

The best information systems often have a gamelike feel. This maxim has been directly translated by people interested in new technology into the development of games and apps that have health-related themes. Games can provoke engagement in users, encouraging self-administration and self-management of chronic diseases. Some games are also designed to reduce stigma, change individuals' self-concept, and enhance self-efficacy (Lieberman, 2012).

A variety of games have been developed for traditional computer and Web platforms, with Facebook especially receiving attention. For example, HealthSeeker is a Facebook game developed in conjunction with the Joslin Diabetes Center. Nintendo's Wii has been used so widely in physical rehabilitation that it has been dubbed "Wii-Hab." Often these games have been developed with the specific input of health professionals. For example, Whyville has content provided by the Centers for Disease Control and is focused on the spread of epidemics.

Increasingly these games are being applied in the area of m-health, with a number of smart phone games. It is estimated that at least 124 million people use smart phones for apps related to such things as logging exercises, tracking blood glucose levels, and even performing ultrasounds. There is almost an endless variety of these games: Elm City Stories aims at encouraging AIDS prevention; Massive Health's Eatery encourages users to lose weight; Quit Now! estimates the money saved for each day someone has quit smoking; and Every Move shares user's activities on Facebook (Dockterman, 2012). In effect, these systems are often intended to link communication and information dosages by matching them to health impacts.

M-health applications have the capacity to reach and follow individuals in real time across the multiple everyday contexts they inhabit in interactive and adaptive ways, with impacts ranging from greater weight loss to greater adherence to scheduled appointments (Riley et al., 2011). So someone who is concerned about nutrition and counting calories can get instantaneous feedback when selecting meals at a new restaurant.

DECISION MAKING

Having too much information can be as problematic as having too little when comparing various health care alternatives (Hibbard, 2003). Adept decision makers know intuitively when they have gathered enough information for any particular purpose. They "satisfice" (MacCrimmon & Taylor, 1976), choosing an alternative that is simply "good enough" rather than optimal. They develop a sense as to when they have spent enough energy searching for information about any problem that confronts them (March, 1994). They also learn to approximate, to judge when they can make a high-enough-quality decision for any particular event (Farace, Monge, & Russell, 1977). Decision makers search for an appropriate solution, not *the* optimal solution (Hickson, 1987). They have developed an appreciation for what their limits are, since they can mentally weigh only so much information at any given time.

Over the last three decades, studies have repeatedly demonstrated that decision making is often an irrational process. In fact, the link between decision making and the processing of information is often much weaker than we would like to believe (Feldman & March, 1981). Decision makers often ask for more information (it is, after all, a part of the decision-making ritual), even when they have sufficient information on hand to make a decision (Klein, 2009). This has direct analogs to the way people can become dependent on drugs and, for some, even on placebo effects.

An interesting paradox in this literature pertains to the relationship between information load and decision making and has direct implications for the matching of appropriate doses. Decision makers often seek more information than needed, even when it induces overload (O'Reilly & Pondy, 1979). While this overload of information decreases decision quality, it increases decision makers' confidence (McKinnon & Bruns, 1992; O'Reilly, Chatham, & Anderson, 1987), satisfaction (O'Reilly, 1980), and consumer comfort (Ward, 1987). Studies of firefighters, horse race handicappers, and weather forecasters show that these experts have increased levels of confidence when they are given more data; yet they typically exhibit worse results (Mauboussin, 2007). The problem is not the sheer amount of data but rather the difficulty in focusing on only the most relevant information. How does an individual determine that he or she should rely on experts, that there is an established body of knowledge? In effect, information becomes very addicting for some individuals; they have a constant desire for more, even when it has harmful effects, with results similar to overdosing on medications.

CONTROLLING THE FLOOD

One central element of our contemporary world is the explosive growth of information, coupled with the ready access instantiated in the Internet. Individuals have to choose from among a variety of information sources. There are literally millions of articles published every year in the technical literature, making it impossible for even the most dedicated individual to keep abreast of developments. For example, it has been calculated that physicians need to read an average of 19 original articles each day to keep abreast of their fields (Choi, 2005). While there are more than 10,000 randomized trials of new intervention approaches every year, very few innovations are ever widely adopted (Grol & Grimshaw, 2003). This overload of information forces decentralization of effort, with increasing responsibility passing to individuals, with their health outcomes often determined by their ability to gather, then intelligently act on, information.

We often struggle, however, with how to transform this information into action. This is most clearly seen in the growing problem with translating research findings into applications in medicine. Audits suggest that across a number of national settings, evidence-based medical practices are not consistently applied. In the face of this glut, some have suggested decentralization may result in more effective distribution of critical information (Su, Huang, & Contractor, 2010).

Information can be defined as any stimulus we register or recognize in the environment around us (Miller, 1969). In this view information involves the recognition of patterns in our surrounding basic matter/energy flows (Bates, 2006; Case, 2012; Farace, Monge, & Russell, 1977; Hjorland, 2007). But there is also a sense that information is what you use to develop a higher level of comfort, perhaps even more of a feeling of familiarity with a situation. The more confident and sure you are about something, the less uncertain it is (Farace, Monge, & Russell, 1977). Thus, information can also be viewed as the number (and perhaps kind) of messages needed to overcome uncertainty (Krippendorf, 1986), and uncertainty reduction has often been cast as a "direct and linear function of an objective quantity of information" (Afifi & Afifi, 2009, p. 1); however, "it is less common but equally important to realize that a surfeit of information can confuse and overwhelm us" (Babrow, Kasch, & Ford, 1998, p. 16).

Classically, information load (or volume in some conceptions [Hurley, Kosenko, & Brashers, 2011]) is seen as a function of the amount and complexity of information. Amount refers to the number of pieces (or bits) of information, somewhat akin to the accumulation of data. Complexity relates to the number of choices or alternatives represented by a stimulus. In a situation where all choices are equally probable, entropy is at its maximum (Farace, Monge, & Russell, 1977). Certainly, in today's world both the amount and complexity of information are increasing nearly exponentially.

On the receiver's side, then, there has been a concern with impacts of communication overloads (Farace, Monge, & Russell, 1977; Fidler & Johnson, 1984; Stohl & Redding, 1987), in part because they can have similar outcomes to overdoses. Disconcertingly, it is also possible that people will become so overloaded with information that they will "escape," turning to demagogues who offer simple solutions to increasingly complex problems. The dark side of the quest for uncertainty reduction is that once an answer is arrived at, a decision made, blockage from future communication may occur (Smithson, 1989).

Denial and escape—that is, refusal to recognize things that are too painful to know—are maladaptive means of adjusting to difficult circumstances and represent major barriers to health communication. It is not uncommon for individuals to avoid information that will force them to make a decision to overcome some problem. It is also common in decision-making situations for individuals to avoid information, to avoid a dose, that conflicts with their chosen course of action (Donohew et al., 1987).

The most basic limit for most of us is time. Even the most trivial tasks could theoretically consume a lifetime, if all the information needed to understand them were gathered. The problem then is not in deciding to seek information but in deciding when to stop. Adept decision makers know intuitively when they have gathered enough information for any particular purpose. They reach these judgments because they have developed an appreciation for what their limits are; they can mentally weigh only so much information at any given time. The ultimate goals of rationality may be to develop a sense of coherence, and a simple one at that, with satisficing as the standard rather than maximizing (Bates, 2005; Pirolli & Card, 1999).

These problems are exacerbated when the uncontrolled flood interacts with other streams or currents that join the river. Instant messaging and peer monitoring, continuous tracking of presence, cause people to lose focus and are distracting, interrupting the flow of work (Cameron & Webster, 2005). Increased connectivity for teleworkers increases stress from interruptions and may indirectly diminish workers identification with their organizations (Fonner & Roloff, 2012). So issues of polychronicity, the superimposition of tasks one on top of another, and multitasking reduce the capacity of individuals to focus on any one problem.

Health professionals' most important role may be as a stimulus or cue to action. They can define the most important issues that the public needs to confront. So attention and agenda setting are the scarce resources, not information; fundamentally we must accept human limits to information processing. Some people have just reached a saturation point; they cannot spend any more time communicating (Fortner, 1995). While more and more information can be produced more efficiently, there is a concomitant increase in the costs of consuming (e.g., interpreting, analyzing) it.

SUMMARY AND COMMENTARY

Table 8.1 summarizes the differences in the dosage elements for the access, facilitating, engagement, decision-making, and flood aspects of health information technology. Access leads to larger amounts, just as facilitating enhances health communication. Engagement encourages receivers and decision makers to strive to gather information that is relevant to a problem. Finally, increased availability leads to the need to control dosage amounts to prevent individuals from being overwhelmed by a deluge of health information.

Frequency is related to increased access and is also promoted by facilitating factors. Engagement stimulates individuals to desire dosages that decision making suggests may be needed to solve particular problems, while monitoring the flood can help to rationalize decision-making processes.

The sequencing of dosages may be blocked in its natural progression, depending on whether or not access is permitted, while facilitating encourages administration of dosages in their proper order. Engagement stimulates the persistence of individuals in administration of doses often meant to affirm that the right decisions have been made. A flood of information may lead to a premature stoppage of searches, while successful regulation of information insures a natural progression of dosages.

Access to a range of delivery systems enhances the possibilities of receiving the right dose and is greatly facilitated by an increased awareness of a variety of options. Although modality switching, say from e-mail to face-to-face, does not necessarily have the intended impact of enhancing intimacy, in part due to expectancy violations (Ramirez & Wang, 2008), often delivery systems that promote a sense of engagement are the most effective ones. Institutions often link delivery systems to software that promotes the sort of

Table 8.1. The Dosage Elements and Health Information Technology

Dosage Elements	Technology				
	Access	Facilitating	Engagement	Decision Making	Flood
Amount	Increasing	Enhancing	Encourage	Relevance	Control
Frequency	Increasing	Promotes	Stimulate	As needed	Monitor
Sequencing	Permits	Encourages	Persistence	Affirmation	Premature Stoppage
Delivery systems	Range	Awareness of	Most effective	Linkage to systems	Efficiency
Interactions	Literacy	Literacy	Demographics	Alternatives	Differential availability
Contraindications	Free access	Cognitive functioning	Self-efficacy	Inexperience	Existing base, multitasking
Dysfunctions	Comprehensability	Overload	Blind enthusiasm	Poor judgment	Paralysis

decision making that we discussed in box 3.3. These systems also often limit the way data can enter the decision-making process and, as a result, help to efficiently manage information.

The elements, such as amount and frequency, often interact with the health literacy levels of individuals. Similarly, different levels of engagement are often produced by channels that are uniquely appealing to members of different demographic groups. So the young are more likely to find Twitter an appealing source of information. The range of alternatives available also influences decision making, and their differential availability can help to manage the flood.

Contraindications and dysfunctions may be associated with free access to information sources that someone is unable to comprehend, producing at the least frustration and potentially leading to critical misunderstandings. Facilitating access can increase information overload, which hampers cognitive functioning. Engagement may lead to erroneous judgments of one's self-efficacy and capability of making decisions that only the most experienced should attempt. Engagement can also produce a blinding enthusiasm that leads to poor judgment. Finally, one's existing information base and capacity for multitasking may be related to whether or not one becomes paralyzed by the flood of potential information one can be exposed to.

We do not have measured approaches to problems. We do not know when to stop, but we are often pressed to do something, to act in the presence of uncertainty, complexity, and a continuing (and growing) stream of knowledge that could easily change our positions. It is obviously impossible for someone to even dream of keeping tabs of everything, even in a very limited domain of knowledge. The question then becomes, How does one control the flood, determining the proper dose and matching the flow of information to one's needs and/or purposes? The consumer movement in medicine assumes individuals are increasingly sophisticated and can understand issues ranging from advanced cell biology to psychosocial adjustment to pain management. Individuals have free access to a world of health information. Our increasingly complex medical systems demand that individuals be able to navigate an often bewildering health care system, and this very capability to navigate becomes an important element of health literacy.

These trends suggest a need to reintroduce simplicity, partially by thinking carefully about what should be excluded from an individual's information processing. While more and more information can be produced more efficiently, there is a concomitant increase in the costs of consuming (e.g., interpreting, analyzing) this information, but, as we have seen, some of the advances in health information technology can help people filter the doses they receive.

FURTHER READINGS

Eysenbach, G. (2005). Design and evaluation of consumer health information Web sites. In D. Lewis, G. Eysenbach, R. Kukafka, P. Z. Stavri & H. B. Jimison (Eds.), *Consumer health informatics: Informing consumers and improving health care* (pp. 34–60). New York: Springer.

Pragmatic discussion of HIT from the perspective of consumer informatics with useful discussion of access.

Johnson, J. D. (2005). *Innovation and knowledge management: The Cancer Information Services Research Consortium*. Cheltenham, UK: Edward Elgar.

An exemplar of the commitment to the development of a national information infrastructure and health information services on the part of the National Institutes of Health.

Walther, J. B., Pingree, S., Hawkins, R. P., & Buller, D. B. (2005). Attributes of interactive online health information systems. *Journal of Medical Internet Research,* 7 (3), E33.

General discussion of key features of health information technology systems.

· 9 ·

Final Analysis

$\mathcal{A}$fter introducing dosage in chapter 1, in the second chapter I focused on unpacking the metaphor of dosage, detailing its many elements, as well as discussing the uses and limits of metaphor generally. The dosage metaphor has broad application to communication across a number of levels of analysis. While a focus on context is certainly convenient and widely accepted, increasingly communication research has found itself divided by its context domains. But beyond this, we may also be divided by our metaphors, with each context appealing to different ones (L. L. Putnam & Boys, 2006). This increasing specialization within communication, as in other disciplines, hinders the development of research in areas like dosage that cut across various contextual domains. Focusing on dosage provides a promise of integrating increasingly fragmented subspecialties within communication.

The most elementary of communication contexts is that focusing on relationships between two people in interpersonal communication. In chapter 3 I focused on physician-patient interactions as an exemplar of a wide range of dyadic relationships where there are asymmetric status and power relationships between health professionals and clients.

Interprofessional teams play an increasingly important role in the delivery of health care. Chapter 4 first discussed the nature of interdisciplinarity and then focused on teamwork, interdependence, frameworks, decision making, and creative problem solving as they relate to the dosage metaphor.

Historically mass media theories such as uses and gratifications, dependency, and the knowledge gap, discussed in chapter 5, have examined issues of exposure and resulting media effects, issues central to any application of dosage to communication phenomenon.

Chapter 6 focused on diffusion and dissemination using the current focus on clinical and translational science as a touchstone. Here I also highlighted network analysis concepts such as the strength of weak ties and social contagion. Chapter 7 then turned to the related issues of the role of communication campaigns in encouraging change in health behaviors. The recent emphasis on health communication has considerably deepened our understanding of campaign effects.

Chapter 8 examined the growing importance of health information technology (HIT). HIT promotes access and facilitates information seeking and resulting decision making, but it also threatens to engulf us in a deluge of information.

In this final chapter I analyze the dosage metaphor in broad sweep and suggest a countervailing minimalist approach to communication before turning to broader policy issues raised by application of the metaphor of dosage as well as detailing its implications for methods of communication research. The chapter concludes with a discussion of the relationship between researchers and practitioners and how dosage can operate as a bridging metaphor to close the gap between these two traditionally separate roles. As we saw in chapter 7, increasingly policy makers, especially in the health field, are resistant to funding research that has no direct practical application.

UNPACKING THE ELEMENTS OF
THE DOSAGE METAPHOR

Metaphors shape how we think about disease, particularly cancer and AIDS (Mukherjee, 2010; Sontag, 1978, 1988). A useful metaphor applies something we know a great deal about to enrich our understanding of its target (Ambrosini, 2003). As we have seen, unpacking the dosage metaphor into its various elements allows us to explore a variety of communication theories in greater depth. These elements often interact with each other in very telling ways. Amount, frequency, and sequencing have separate but strongly interrelated impacts, so one is instructed to take a five milligram drug five times a day, and either two hours before or after eating. The possible combinations expand nearly exponentially with each additional drug one takes.

Communication theories seldom are this sophisticated,[1] although increasingly media, political, and marketing campaigns are becoming very targeted in their reach to their audiences based on dollar-value return for delivery systems ranging from robo calls to ubiquitous television commercials to door-to-door canvasing. Increasingly HMOs and other larger health organizations are using similar techniques involving health information technology, especially for reminders related to screening tests.

For delivery systems, as in these campaigns, there is an awareness of the differential impacts of various communication channels, although mass media and interpersonal scholars have often been criticized for establishing a synthetic competition in their theorizing (Chaffee, 1979). Delivery systems also imply sophisticated understanding of the most efficacious ways of delivering treatment agents. The work of pharmacists is often centered on more appropriate ways of delivering treatment agents, ranging from nasal sprays for those who resist having shots to reformulated therapeutic agents for those who cannot take them orally.

Interactions and contraindications can both temper the impacts of dosages. When a dose interacts with another factor, it is changed in various ways. So, if I am conducting a face-to-face communication campaign in conjunction with changes in laws, such as those related to smoking in public places, change will be greatly reinforced.

Contraindications indicate situations where a dose might produce a more deleterious outcome than intended. Perhaps because the potential for the dark side in communication is seldom seriously examined in communication theories, there is less of an understanding of these issues in communication. So assurances that a crisis situation is something that the public need not worry about, when an institution knows that there is a problem, while having a short-term benefit, can lead to disastrous long-term consequences for the organization that might be more problematic than immediately having admitted it.

Similarly, the dysfunctional impacts of dosages have also received minimal attention. So a manager who answers every employee's query with a sympathetic ear and nurturing response may in the long run be creating a dependent relationship, just as a helicopter parent does, where the employee becomes incapable of autonomous action. Similarly, it is now widely understood that teams and ad hoc groups, while useful when an organization is confronted with an uncertain environment where new or novel responses are needed, can be a dysfunctional waste of resources in situations of low uncertainty, where routines have been established.

EVALUATING THE DOSAGE METAPHOR AS A THEORY-BUILDING DEVICE

> Now biologists, having absorbed the methods and vocabulary of communication science, went further to make their own contributions to the understanding of information itself (Gleick, 2011, p. 310).

As this quote suggests, application of the dosage metaphor can be a two-way street, with both sides learning about the problems they are interested in. I have attempted here to uncover the pervasiveness of the dosage metaphor in prior thinking about communication to reveal that it is tacitly conventionalized in many theories of communication, especially those focusing on issues of intimacy, exposure, and change.

There are numerous ways we can evaluate theory. Certainly dosage has been widely used as a means for predicting, explaining, and controlling health. It offers a number of tools that could be widely applied to communication problems, such as the dose-response curve and therapeutic index. In that sense it could be very appealing as a generative device for enriching our understanding of communication, focusing our attention on a variety of new ways of approaching our task. In this way the application of metaphor can provide us with an "imaginative rationality" (Lakoff & Johnson, 1980). At a naive level, all of us understand dose. Hopefully this work has demonstrated there are multiple manifestations of dosage in a variety of communication contexts and theories and that thinking about communication with this metaphor rings true and resonates (Mangham, 1996).

On its face, dosage is a simple, elegant, and parsimonious way of heuristically approaching communication problems and issues. However, it may not be aesthetically appealing to many because of its strong roots in medical approaches and its linkage to administrative science. This, when coupled with its linear, top-down feel for many who have a relatively naive understanding of the metaphor, may result in a near visceral reaction to its application to communication. But, for example, nurses, much like effective communication practitioners, continue to monitor the impacts of dosages on patients and receive feedback, adjusting treatments in conjunction with others on the treatment team.

The study of the metaphor can enrich the understanding of both the phenomenon to which it is applied and the underlying metaphor itself. What can communication scholars contribute to our understanding of dosage in medicine? Perhaps our greatest contribution can come in greater understanding of audience reaction/receptivity issues, which is central to the application of personalized medicine in genomics. How a message is perceived really determines the nature of a communication event, with receivers ultimately determining its meaning (Hall, 1981; Rowley & Turner, 1978). It is the audience that ultimately interprets any message (Morley, 1993) and, more basically, determines whether any communication will occur (Katz, Blumler, & Gurevitch, 1974).

As the classic selective perception and selective attention literatures suggest (Katz, 1968), a fundamental property of communication relationships is that a receiver must attend to a communication message for any communication to occur (Drucker, 1974). In a somewhat similar way, one of the fundamental understudied problems of medical approaches is that patients often administer dosages in ways that diminish their impact because of costs, side effects, and so on. Even more interestingly, in the study of nocebo effects, how a treatment is framed may determine individuals' reactions to it. So, if chemotherapy is seen as having devastating side effects, many patients will experience them, even if the medication does not biologically produce them.

In the end, the dosage metaphor may be much more appealing than a variety of alternative candidates that have been proposed as encompassing metaphors for communication, including container, conduit, transmission, control, war, and dance (Krippendorf, 1993). This may be especially so in joint projects involving researchers and practitioners. Hopefully, I have demonstrated that the dosage metaphor allows us to see things in a new light and then easily communicate them to others, thus allowing us to communicate more effectively, providing an interpretive framework, a common ground, for the other and an encompassing framework for theory and research.

A MINIMALIST APPROACH TO COMMUNICATION

Information has always been a source of power, but it is now increasingly a source of confusion. In every sphere of modern life, the chronic condition is a surfeit of information, poorly integrated or lost somewhere in the system (Wilensky, 1968, p. 331).

All too often the problem is *not* that the two sides do not understand each other and that this misunderstanding generates conflict. No, often the two sides *do* clearly understand each other, and the recognition of the other's possible gain at their expense causes the strife. As one rather cynical student activist put it, "It's not a lack of communication that's causing the problem. In fact, if we knew more about why they were doing it, it would probably make us *more* militant rather than less!" Communications may help, but it is usually not enough to resolve genuine conflicts of interest. The "communication fallacy" must be avoided, if we are to understand the political dynamics of conflict (Baldridge, 1971, pp. 202, italics in the original).

"It is the dose that makes a poison," runs an old adage in medicine (Mukherjee, 2010, p. 143).

Traditionally, it has been argued that the way to improve organizations is not to produce more information but to reduce the amount of information any one subsystem must process (March & Simon, 1958). Increasingly the ability to focus and to develop coherent approaches to an increasingly complex world may be the most useful approach. As we have noted, Hansen and Haas (2001) found an interesting paradox in knowledge markets: the less information a supplier provided, the more it was used, because of a reputation the supplier developed for focus and quality. Indeed, lower levels of face-to-face communication had many positive impacts for teleworkers: fewer distractions, less involvement in office politics, and greater job satisfaction (Fonner & Roloff, 2010).

As I noted at the outset of this work, there has been a communication metamyth that more is necessarily better. As a result we do not have measured approaches to problems. We do not know when to stop, and perhaps like a doctor who gives someone a drug because he or she expects one, we are often pressed to do something. What is our equivalent of the "effective dose" concept in medicine—the smallest amount of a substance needed to produce a measurable effect? It has been suggested that one approach to designing interventions would be to start with the minimal intervention needed for change, and only when this proved to be unsuccessful should we proceed to more expensive, complicated interventions (Glasgow, Marcus, et al., 2004).

It has been argued that attention rather than information is the scarcest resource (Pirolli & Card, 1999; Simon, 1987; A. H. Van de Ven, 1986)[2]; fundamentally we must accept human limits to information processing. Although more and more information can be produced more efficiently, there is a concomitant increase in the costs of consuming (e.g., interpreting, analyzing) it (More, 1990).

These trends suggest a need to reintroduce simplicity and to think carefully about what information should be excluded. Knowledge disavowal is indeed important; it allows for the dismissal of disconfirming ideas and the recognition of ideas as not fully formed, at least not developed enough to overturn conventional wisdom, and it is one way of coping with information overload (Zaltman, 1994). How we go about forgetting is becoming a critical issue (Argote, 1999; Argote & Epple, 1990; Govindarajan & Trimble, 2005), as we are continually being asked to process an overwhelming flood of information.

IMPLICATIONS FOR METHODS

One implication of a focus on dosage is a much more serious and rigorous approach to research.[3] While it has become unfashionable to adopt methods from the "harder" sciences, looking closely at what they have done at least acquaints us with some pitfalls and major issues.[4] It also highlights some continuing problems with "business as usual," the state-of-the-art in communication research. First, most of our statistical analyses have a taken-for-granted assumption of linear effects, not the curvilinear ones associated with optimal dosages and with the fundamental issue of match. Second, our measurement techniques do not have the rigorous underlying metrics and associated mathematical properties that the notion of dosage would seem to require. We do not have theoretically driven measures (Epstein & Street, 2007). Further, do we know, as in nutrition, what is really causing the impact, what the active ingredients are? Dosage may be the ultimate variable—since its very essence is in variance. Third, we haven't come to grips with longitudinal effects of the sort needed to assess issues like tolerance, flushing, absorption, and cumulative toxic effects, in spite of a near growth industry in calls for longitudinal research. We have nothing like a dose-response curve or the bioavailability formula,[5] which are well understood in pharmaceutical applications and are very important in determining safe versus hazardous levels of dosages for drugs.[6] So, current m-health applications are based on intraindividual tailoring and just-in-time interventions, rather than classic between-subject considerations, and could benefit from the application of dosage methods (Riley et al., 2011).

Recently, partially because of the advent of the Internet, randomized trials have been compromised, because of the ethical problems of some patients serving as controls, sharing of knowledge, and talking back, all problems that have historically plagued research in organizations. Much like patient advocacy groups that press for the actual treatment, what organization in trouble is going to stand for being a control? In this later sense, negotiating with the subjects of research, the organizational communication research community may have something to offer the biomedical community in the sort of interactive dialog that some have suggested more modern approaches to metaphor should have (Cornelissen, 2005).

What is our version of clinical trials? We simply do not have the underlying science of randomized clinical trials upon which to base prescriptions, in spite of recent suggestions that we should move to evidence-based management (Pfeffer & Sutton, 2006; Rousseau & McCarthy, 2007). To say the least, it is difficult to conduct rigorous experiments because of naturalism—the lack of cumulative effects, clutter-message competition, selective exposure, and so on (Slater, 2004). Dose-response problems require more sophisticated propensity models to deal with complicated interactions in exposure (Slater, 2004), and there has been some recent movement, particularly at Ohio State University, to develop new approaches. On the other hand, there have been at best a handful of organizational studies—some would suggest none (Reay, Berta, & Kahn, 2009)—that have had the rigorous double-blind, randomized control trials needed to test the efficacy of a drug. In addition, somewhat similarly to drug testing (e.g., lack of testing on all but pregnant women, children, and the elderly), we do not apply our research to a range of settings, relying for the most part on convenience samples.

We don't even meet the most rudimentary requirements for scientific rigor in most communication contexts, especially when the potential consequences are considered (e.g., what malpractice insurer would cover a consultant who could conceivably bankrupt a firm?). Do we have a version of drug recall when harmful effects for our interventions are uncovered?

IMPLICATIONS FOR POLICY

One key issue that any policy maker in this area must confront is, Do we really know what end state is desirable? With medicine, we can always argue better health. However, for communication issues this may not be as clear-cut. In chapter 3 we discussed the ideology of openness and its influence on interpersonal communication. This ideology led to recommendations regarding self-disclosure that were later demonstrated to be harmful to the very relationships they aimed to help. So the natural suggestion that we want honesty as the ultimate end state of relationships proved troubling. We have also had suggestions, particularly in the realm of administrative research in communication campaigns, that we should manipulate messages to achieve pronounced impacts since we know what's good for people. However, there have been enough examples now of campaigns, such as breast self-examination, that had well-intentioned goals and were successful but actually resulted in harm to the targeted individuals.

So the question remains, What should be the ultimate goal? What outcome would we like to achieve from a greater understanding of the dosage metaphor in communication? Perhaps the simplest, most unifying goal, one that everyone might rally around, is greater fidelity between what the receiver intends in the message and what is actually received, even if it does not result in compliance. In other words, we seek to achieve higher levels of understanding of the communication messages that we exchange with others. In pursuing this goal we are confronted with the limits of receivers' processing ability and various ethical problems.

Innumeracy

While there has been great public concern with growing illiteracy, there is also a substantial, often hidden problem with innumeracy. This is most clearly manifested in the public's difficulty in analyzing the risk associated with various health procedures, particularly involving dosages of medicine (Epstein & Street, 2007; Rifkin & Bouwer, 2007). Metaphors might be particularly useful ways of attacking the difficulties inherent in communicating risks (Turner, Skubisz, & Rimal, 2011). However, there is a growing cultural indifference, and at times (especially academically) hostility, to numbers. This is fed somewhat by the societal reaction to quants and their role in the hedge fund debacle and the resulting recent financial meltdown, as well as the generalized perception that there are lies, damn lies, and then statistics.

There also has been a growing concern with how risk is communicated to the public, with health communication campaigns and media stories in particular likely to mislead the public about its level of risk, creating an illusion of certainty (Rifkin & Bouwer, 2007). The rise of health consumerism can exacerbate the difficulties that result. The way risk is framed can produce considerably different impacts. There is a clear tendency for people to accept risks associated with medicines when information is presented positively, in terms of increased probability of survival, for example, as opposed to negatively, such as a greater risk of dying (Epstein & Street, 2007).

Dose-response assessments concerning identified hazards result in an overall risk characterization that in turn results in risk-management decisions (Rifkin & Bouwer, 2007). The dose-response assessment answers the question, What is the relationship between the agent and potential adverse health effects? Good dose-response information permits one to scientifically calculate health risk and particular levels of exposure. This is typically important in assessing the impact of carcinogens, where small doses may have no adverse effect (Rifkin & Bouwer, 2007). However, there is a tendency for people to believe that such harmful agents are inherently bad, not to appreciate the concept of an acceptable risk (Rifkin & Bouwer, 2007; B. Schwartz, 2004).

Ethical Issues

A wide variety of ethical and/or dysfunctional issues are associated with the dosage metaphor. They also assist us in understanding the darker side of communication relationships. Often dysfunctional views emerge when a metaphor is explored at a deeper level. So one may start out with a surface metaphor of an organization as one big happy family and only on deeper reflection uncover family feuds, sibling rivalry, nepotism, and in-law relationships (L. L. Putnam & Boys, 2006), with some suggesting that mergers and acquisitions are best understood through a stepfamily metaphor (Allred, Boal, & Holstein, 2005).

Communication as a field has paid little attention to issues of its lingering impacts. While the necessity of flushing out harmful drugs is widely recognized in pharmaceutical applications, it has received scant attention within our field.[7] This is also true for issues relating to the creation of dependent relationships. Can communication be addictive? Do we have the equivalent of detox programs?

Some treatments mask symptoms, so soaring rhetoric can substitute for real action, delaying needed problem confrontation. Organizations can substitute symbols for action. This is often the case for symbolic participation in innovations not because they are necessarily needed or desirable but because they demonstrate to external stakeholders that you are riding the wave of current trends. This is particularly true of information technology and the current fascination of universities with distance learning programs.

An enhanced understanding of dosage impacts offers the real possibility of manipulating audiences. Unfortunately in the commercial world of marketing and the political world of voter turnout and suppression, very sophisticated dosage applications already exist, but they are proprietary. One of the great public policy issues of our times is related to the financing of political campaigns and equating them to "free" speech issues. If not everyone has access to the same possibilities for delivering messages (e.g., buying air time for commercials), what does this mean for our public discourse? Uncovering and making transparent these impacts would make for more sophisticated audiences who might be better able to resist the dark side.

A NEW BRIDGING METAPHOR FOR RESEARCHERS AND PRACTITIONERS

> The knowledge that researchers, teachers, consultants, and practitioners learn by themselves is different and partial. If it could be co-produced and combined in some novel ways the results could produce a dazzling synthesis that could profoundly advance theory, teaching, and practice (A. Van de Ven, 2000, p. 5).

> Metaphors are not only important as tools for intellectual analysis, but offer a unifying vehicle through which academics and audiences can better understand each other (Varan, 1998, p. 59).

Often academic research has not focused on the goal of usefulness, and as a result it has typically not had an impact on practice (D. L. Shapiro, Kirkman, & Courtney, 2007), in spite of growing cries for evidence-based practice. Because of the lack of evidence-based approaches to pragmatic problems, we are often placed in the position of the proverbial country doctor who treats patients more on the basis of art and accumulated experience. Often the critical impact of this relationship is a placebo effect, which results from the trust and faith of the patient in the doctor. However, following the medical model, powerful medicines, with documented scientific impacts, may need certified, licensed practitioners to administer them, with some doses and agents considered illegal (e.g., antitrust, mistreatment of others, intimidation, harassment).[8]

One could even ask whether our current state of knowledge would make it possible for us to create professions like dosimetrist, one of the currently hot health care jobs (Wolgemuth, 2009). A dosimetrist is a member of a radiation oncology team responsible for calculating and measuring the dose of radiation that will be used for treatment. Do we have the mind-set to prepare communication students to become practitioners by giving them tools to approach the problems they confront in the same manner?

The possibility of bridging the divide between researchers and practitioners has been a recurring theme of leaders in a variety of academic disciplines (Applegate, 2001, 2002; P. Cullen et al., 2001; A. Van de Ven, 2000, 2002), with some suggesting metaphors can be essential to achieving this end (Kent, 2001). It has also been noted that even for applied subfields, such as health communication, the greatest shortcoming of academic research is its lack of relevance to practitioners, its inability to be translated (Babrow & Mattson, 2003; Dorsey, 2003; T. L. Thompson, 2003). Indeed, the issue of translation, as we have seen from chapter 6, from bench to bedside, has become central to the work of the National Institutes of Health, in part because of growing pressure from Congress. The history of the development of dosage also contains an implicit division of labor between researchers and practitioners, one that also provides a bridging metaphor between groups that seem to grow further apart with each passing year.

In general, for researchers, there are considerable benefits that can ensue from interacting with practitioners; in fact, they may have more to gain from researcher-practitioner relationships (RPR) than do practitioners. While both parties have things to gain from RPRs, they often have even more to lose. Both parties have substantial potential common benefits from a successful RPR, including securing both physical and material resources and intellectual stimulation (P. W. Cullen et al., 1999). It is also obvious that policy makers see substantial benefits to be had from interactions between the various parties in the research enterprise, with increasing calls from the National Cancer Institute (2003) and the Fund for the Improvement of Postsecondary Education (2003), among others, for holistic examinations of research problems through the development of synergistic relationships among often fractured disciplines (Wandersman, Goodman, & Butterfoss, 1997). Many have suggested that a richer intellectual synergy can develop from combining theory and practice, resulting in greater understanding and a more comprehensive view of phenomena of interest. We have tended to focus on knowledge transfer, rather than knowledge production, in making our research relevant to practitioners (D. L. Shapiro, Kirkman, & Courtney, 2007); in doing this we have implicitly argued that we know what's best for them. One potential benefit of the dosage metaphor is that it provides a common point of orientation for both researchers and practitioners—a theme they can play off.

Some have suggested that the lack of utilization of social science findings by practitioners and policy makers is essentially attributable to their different frames—they have conflicting values, different reward systems, and different languages (Kuhn, 2002; Reay, Berta, & Kahn, 2009). These obstacles are always difficult to overcome, especially as they relate to continuing unfilled manifest needs (e.g., publications, improved practice) of the parties.

While both parties have things to gain from the RPR, they often have even more to lose, which can lead to difficulties in maintaining relationships and even their eventual dissolution (J. D. Johnson, 2004). One of the paramount values of any science is the objectivity of researchers and the preservation of their ability to maintain their independence and integrity. Often practitioners, by questioning some taken-for-granted assumptions, threaten researchers' autonomy in ways that call into question these fundamental principles. Practitioners seldom have any great concern for the integrity of the research process, especially relating to traditional scientific verities associated with rigorous research and internal validity (Kilmann, Slevin, & Thomas, 1983). They will change interventions if they sense they are not working to the benefit of their project, since this is, after all, what they do daily in their operations. "Because sponsors' needs come first, program improvement second, and evaluator's needs are only a third priority, in many evaluation studies you'll have little control over the evaluation itself and none, typically, over the object of evaluation" (J. Dearing, May 2000, p. 8). Practitioners also may not respect researcher's needs for confidentiality of privileged scientific information, thus interfering with patent, publication, and other intellectual property rights (Keen & Stocklmayer, 1999).

Relationships with practitioners can also be very threatening to researchers' self-concepts. First, as Goodall (1989) has demonstrated, researchers are often manipulated by skilled practitioners so that these practitioners can achieve their own ends. Second, critique from practitioners often centers around two opposing themes of common sense or naiveté: either "you're not telling us anything we do not already know," or your ideas are so "pie in the sky," or abstract, that they could never work. Since these judgments are often based on professional experience and anecdote, they are not easily refutable. They also may be quite telling; since we often seek to describe the world as it is, we lag behind real-world events and often merely describe the experience of a skilled practitioner. So, practitioners often feel researchers are out of touch with real-world practices (Ford et al., 2003; Rynes, Bartunek, & Daft, 2001), a critical shortcoming in this fast-moving world. Similarly, in our quest for methodological rigor, we often ignore variables, especially political and legal ones, that any practitioner must consider before implementing a new practice. Paradoxically, the more sophisticated our methods and theories, the less useful they appear to practitioners (Rynes, Bartunek, & Daft, 2001) and, ironically, the less likely they are to produce findings of powerful effects (Hornik, 2002a). We cannot just throw up our arms and say that communication is so complex that we cannot achieve the level of science of simple medicines—practitioners will still confront these problems on a daily basis and prescribe remedies.

One interesting feature of RPRs is that it is quite possible for one party to achieve his or her goals while the overall system fails. So an innovation might be adopted that benefits practitioners, but the research is so commonplace, or flawed because of lack of rigor, that it is not diffused through the academic literature. A true partnership with practitioners is very time-consuming, and the resulting rewards are typically slight, since these partnerships are seldom valued institutionally (Keen & Stocklmayer, 1999).

More disturbingly, often a failed project results in interesting research. Herein lies a clear challenge for researchers. Often we learn as much or more from failed efforts we are involved in as from successful ones. So our own individual goals are likely to be achieved regardless of the outcomes of the overall project. And we can often take comfort in the fact that we preserved the canons of our profession. Unfortunately citation analyses also indicate that relationships in which researchers define the problems and pursue their own questions are most likely to be successful in academic terms (Rynes, Bartunek, & Daft, 2001). So in some ways you have the paradox of success: the more successful one entity in a system is in attaining its more limited individual goals, the more unlikely it is that the overall system will attain its wider objective (Senge, 1990).

This leads to the troubling question of who's responsibility it really is to ensure that what researchers learn is actually distributed to practice (Glasgow et al., 2004)—if we build it, they won't necessarily come. The answers to these questions pose important issues for policy makers within the National Cancer Institute (2003), who are increasingly focused on how best to translate all of their research products into practice. All this is perhaps most poignantly summarized in the following quote from a report of an extremely well-funded researcher:

> Although such research could make important contributions to the science of cancer prevention and control, sustaining interventions like the one tested here is of major concern. At the present time, there would seem to be few organizations prepared to adopt this type of intervention beyond the research setting (Marcus et al., 2001, p. 213).

CONCLUSION

Ultimately a metaphor works or it does not; its beauty is in the eye of the beholder. Hopefully I have demonstrated that the dosage metaphor has historically permeated communication research and theory and that it is a strong metaphor that is markedly emphatic and resonant (Black, 1979). Greater appreciation of its centrality can help us advance health communication, while also making us more relevant to the world of practice. Communication purists who resist reducing the complexities of communication to a formula should understand the frustration that this produces in practitioners and how they will cope with it. If we do not respond to their needs, they will turn to others who offer them facile solutions because the problems are compelling and they need to act. Our lack of methodological sophistication should cause communication researchers to pause, both in terms of our limited understanding of the processes really operative in our understanding of dosage and in terms of the potential consequences of the application of our limited understanding if applied in real-world settings. As this book reveals, the study of dosage can be deep and rich, offering a wealth of possible approaches to problems and a bridge to fractured subspecialties within communication, as well as to the world of practice.

NOTES

1. The issue of amount and frequency in terms of building up to a certain level of critical mass has been rigorously detailed in some network analysis approaches.

2. In their highly influential study of university presidents, Cohen and March (1986) suggest that one basic problem for universities and their leaders is a failure to identify a satisfactory metaphor for how they function.

3. One could hope that this might follow the pattern found for contemporary network analysis, which has moved from a powerful metaphor to a set of sophisticated analytic techniques (Breiger, 2004).

4. Amazon.com has over a thousand results for books on dosage calculations in medicine.

5. Although there are some similarities to the classic S-curve in diffusion, it is most often used in a more descriptive than predictive sense.

6. However, we need not limit ourselves to just quantitative approaches to dosage-related issues. The narrative turn in communication (Fisher, 1987; Sharf & Vanderford, 2003; T. L. Thompson, 2003), itself a metaphor, suggests that compelling stories are the best means of advancing a discipline. By understanding stories and metaphors, we come to grips with the generative mechanisms that drive human action in particular contexts and provide explanations for why things happened in

certain ways (Sharf & Vanderford, 2003). The continuing fascination of the television audience with medical dramas like *House* relates to a search for the right agents and the right dosages of them to confront time-dependent problems (while House himself is searching for the right dosage of various medicines to manage his own pain [D. O. Case, personal communication, April 7, 2007]). Health communicators face these issues every day, providing us with an underlying narrative thread with which to understand their basic approach to decision making.

7. We do not have Darwinian approaches to our ideas, which all still may be in place somewhere. In other words, do we have any mechanism for eliminating the old? Just as physicians seldom learn new tricks once they leave school, in spite of licensing that depends on continuing education, there are many professors who teach for a generation without ever escaping their past.

8. An early torture method of European fascists was to overdose their victims with castor oil. As many have unfortunately discovered, end-of-life treatments (e.g., chemotherapy, radical surgery) often lead to worse outcomes than reasoned acceptance of one's fate.

FURTHER READINGS

Krippendorf, K. (1993). Major metaphors of communication and some constructivist reflections on their use. *Cybernetics and Human Knowing, 2* (1), 3–25.

Explores the use of metaphor in constructing scientific communication theories and communication more generally as a social phenomenon. This article discusses the various metaphors that have been applied to the field of communication in general, including container, conduit, transmission, control, war, and dance. Krippendorf argues that we cannot think of communication without them.

Marshak, R. J. (1996). Metaphors, metaphoric fields and organizational change. In D. Grant & C. Oswick (Eds.), *Metaphor and organizations* (pp. 147–165). Thousand Oaks, CA: Sage.

Discusses systematically how metaphors can be analyzed by their depth, breadth, interrelationships, and coherence.

Reay, T., Berta, W., & Kahn, M. K. (2009). What's the evidence on evidence-based management? *Academy of Management Perspectives, 23* (4), 5–18.

A discomforting analysis of how much evidence we really have to apply to practice in the area of management.

Bibliography

Abbott, A. (1981). Status and strain in the professions. *American Journal of Sociology*, *86*, 819–835.

Abbott, A. (1988). *The system of professions: An essay on the division of expert labor.* Chicago: University of Chicago Press.

Abelson, R. P. (1964). Mathematical models of the distribution of attitudes under controversy. In N. Frederiksen & H. Gulliksen (Eds.), *Contributions to mathematical psychology* (pp. 141–164). New York: Holt, Rinehart, and Winston.

Abigail, R. A., & Cahn, D. D. (2013). Working with you is killing me: Learning how to effectively handle workplace conflict. In J. S. Wrench (Ed.), *Workplace communication in the 21st century: Tools and strategies that impact the bottom line* (pp. 289–319). Santa Barbara, CA: Praeger.

Adams, J. S. (1980). Interorganizational processes and organizational activities. In S. B. Bacharach (Ed.), *Research in organizational behavior* (Vol. 2, pp. 321–355). Greenwich, CT: JAI Press.

Adelman, M. B., Parks, M. R., & Albrecht, T. L. (1987). Beyond close relationships: Support in weak ties. In T. L. Albrecht & M. B. Adelman (Eds.), *Communicating social support* (pp. 126–147). Newbury Park, CA: Sage.

Afifi, T. D., & Afifi, W. A. (2009). Introduction. In T. D. Afifi & W. A. Afifi (Eds.), *Uncertainty, information management, and disclosure decisions: Theories and applications* (pp. 1–5). New York: Routledge.

Afifi, W. (2009). Uncertainty management theories. In S. W. Littlejohn & K. A. Foss (Eds.), *Encyclopedia of communication theory* (Vol. 2, pp. 973–976). Los Angeles: Sage.

Agrell, A., & Gustafson, R. (1996). Innovation and creativity in work groups. In M. West (Ed.), *Handbook of work group psychology* (pp. 317–343). Sussex, UK: John Wiley.

Ahuja, G. (2000). Collaboration networks, structural holes, and innovation: A longitudinal study. *Administrative Science Quarterly*, *45*, 425–455.

Ajzen, I. (1985). From intentions to actions: A theory of planned behavior. In J. Kuhl & J. Beckmann (Eds.), *Action-control: From cognition and behavior* (pp. 11–39). Heidelberg, Germany: Springer.

Ajzen, I. (1987). Attitudes, traits, and actions: Dispositional prediction of behavior in personality and social psychology. *Advances in Experimental Social Psychology, 20*, 1–63.

Ajzen, I., & Fishbein, M. (1980). *Understanding attitudes and predicting social behavior*. Englewood Cliffs, NJ: Prentice Hall.

Albrecht, T. L. (1982). Coping with occupational stress: Relational and individual strategies of nurses in acute health care settings. In M. Burgoon (Ed.), *Communication yearbook 6* (pp. 832–849). Beverly Hills, CA: Sage.

Albrecht, T. L., & Adelman, M. B. (1987a). Communicating social support: A theoretical perspective. In T. L. Albrecht & M. B. Adelman (Eds.), *Communication social support* (pp. 18–39). Newbury Park, CA: Sage.

Albrecht, T. L., & Adelman, M. B. (1987b). Communication networks as structures of social support. In T. L. Albrecht & M. B. Adelman (Eds.), *Communicating social support* (pp. 40–63). Newbury Park, CA: Sage.

Albrecht, T. L., & Adelman, M. B. (1987c). Rethinking the relationship between communication and social support: An introduction. In T. L. Albrecht & M. B. Adelman (Eds.), *Communicating social support* (pp. 13–16). Newbury Park, CA: Sage.

Albrecht, T. L., & Hall, B. (1989). *Relational and content differences between elites and outsiders in innovation networks*. Paper presented at the Annual Meetings of the International Communication Association Convention, San Francisco, CA.

Albrecht, T. L., Irey, K. V., & Mundy, A. K. (1982). Integration in communication networks as a mediator of stress: The case of a protective services agency. *Social Work, 27*, 225–236.

Allred, B. B., Boal, K. B., & Holstein, W. K. (2005). Corporations as stepfamilies: A new metaphor for explaining the fate of merged and acquired companies. *Academy of Management Executive, 19* (3), 23–37.

Altman, I., & Taylor, D. A. (1973). *Social penetration: The development of interpersonal relationships*. New York: Holt, Rinehart and Winston.

Amabile, T. M., Patterson, C., Mueller, J., Wojcik, T., Odomirok, P. W., Marsh, M. M., & Kramer, S. J. (2001). Acadamic-practitioner collaboration in management research: A case of cross-profession collaboration. *Academy of Management Journal, 44*, 418–431.

Ambrosini, V. (2003). *Tacit and ambiguous resources as sources of competitive advantage*. New York: Palgrave MacMillan.

Anderson, L. N., & Walsch, D. L. (2013). Every organization faces risk, but effectively communicating risks is a skill. In J. S. Wrench (Ed.), *Workplace communication for the 21st century: Tools and strategies that impact the bottom line* (Vol. 2, pp. 215–234). Santa Barbara, CA: Praeger.

Andrews, J. E., Johnson, J. D., Case, D. O., Allard, S. L., & Kelley, K. (2005). Intention to seek information on cancer genetics. *Information Research, 10*.

Andrykowski, M. A., Lightner, R., Studts, J. L., & Munn, R. K. (1997). Hereditary cancer risk notification and testing: How interested is the general population. *Journal of Clinical Oncology, 15*, 2139–2148.

Andrykowski, M. A., Munn, R. K., & Studts, J. L. (1996). Interest in learning of a personal genetic predisposition for cancer: Results of a general population survey. *Preventive Medicine, 25*, 527–536.

Ansari, S. M., Fiss, P. C., & Zajac, E. J. (2010). Made to fit: How practices vary as they diffuse. *Academy of Management Review, 35* (1), 67–92.

Applegate, J. L. (2001). Engaged graduate education: Skating to where the puck will be. *Spectra, 37*, 1–5.

Applegate, J. L. (2002). Skating to where the puck will be: Engaged research as a funding strategy for the communication discipline. *Journal of Applied Communication Research, 30*, 402–410.

Argote, L. (1999). *Organizational learning: Creating, retaining and transferring knowledge.* Boston: Kluwer Academic Publishers.

Argote, L., & Epple, D. (1990). Learning curves in manufacturing. *Science, 247*, 920–924.

Armenakis, A. A., & Bedeian, A. G. (1992). The role of metaphors in organizational change: Change agent and change target perspectives. *Group and Organization Management, 17*, 242–248. doi: 10.1177/1059601192173003.

Armstrong, K., Schwartz, J. S., & FitzGerald, G. (2002). Effect of framing as gain vs. loss on hypothetical treatment choices: Survival and mortality curves. *Medical Decision Making, 21*, 76–83.

Armstrong, K., Weber, B., Ubel, P. A., Guerra, C., & Schwartz, J. S. (2002). Interest in BRCA 1/2 testing in a primary care population. *Preventive Medicine, 34*, 590–595. doi: 10.1006/pmed.2002.1022.

Ashford, S. J., Blatt, R., & VandeWalle, D. (2003). Reflections on the looking glass: A review of research on feedback seeking behavior in organizations. *Journal of Management, 29*, 773–799.

Atkin, C. (1979). Research evidence on mass mediated health communication campaigns. In D. Nimmo (Ed.), *Communication yearbook 3*. New Brunswick, NJ: Transaction Books.

Atkin, C. K. (1981). Mass communication research principles for health education. In M. Meyer (Ed.), *Health education by television and radio: Contributions to an international conference with a selected bibliography* (pp. 41–55). New York: K. G. Saur.

Averbeck, J. M., Jones, A., & Robertson, K. (2011). Prior knowledge and health messages: An examination of affect as heuristics and information as systematic processing for fear appeals. *Southern Communication Journal, 76* (1), 35–54. doi: 10.1080/10417940902951824.

Avins, M. (2000a, August 7). Genome map success: Much yet to discover. *Los Angeles Times.* Retrieved from http://web.lexis-nexis.com/universe/document?_ansett=GeHauKO-.

Avins, M. (2000b, July 27). Los Angeles Time Poll. *Los Angeles Times.* Retrieved from http://web.lexis-nexis.com/universe/document?_ansett=GeHauKO-.

Aydin, C. E., Ball-Rokeach, S. J., & Reardon, K. K. (1991). *Mass media resources for social comparison among breast cancer patients.* Paper presented at the International Communication Association, Chicago, IL.

Ayme, S., Kole, A., & Groft, S. (2008). Empowerment of patients: Lessons from the rare disease community. *Lancet, 371,* 2048–2051.

Babrow, A. S. (2001). Guest editor's introduction to the special issue on uncertainty, evaluation, and communication. *Journal of Communication, 51,* 453–455.

Babrow, A. S., Kasch, C. R., & Ford, L. A. (1998). The many meanings of uncertainty in illness: Toward a systematic accounting. *Health Communication, 10* (1), 1–23.

Babrow, A. S., & Mattson, M. (2003). Theorizing about health communication. In T. L. Thompson, A. M. Dorsey, K. I. Miller & R. Parrott (Eds.), *Handbook of health communication* (pp. 35–61). Mahwah, NJ: Lawrence Erlbaum Associates.

Baldridge, J. V. (1971). *Power and conflict in the University: Research in the sociology of complex organizations.* New York: John Wiley.

Balkundi, P., & Harrison, D. A. (2006). Ties, leaders, and time in teams: Strong inference about network structure's effect on team viability and performance. *Academy of Management Journal, 49,* 49–68.

Ball-Rokeach, S. J., & DeFleur, M. L. (1976). A dependency model of mass media effects. *Communication Research, 1,* 3–21.

Banas, J. A., & Rains, S. A. (2010). A meta-analysis of research on inoculation theory. *Commuication Monographs, 77* (3), 281–311. doi: 10.1080/03637751003758193.

Bandolier. (2004). Patient compliance with satins. *Bandolier.* Retrieved from http://www.medicine.ox.ac.uk/bandolier/booth/cardiac/patcomp.html.

Barak, A., Boniel-Nissim, M., & Suler, J. (2008). Fostering empowerment in online support groups. *Computers in Human Behavior, 24,* 1867–1883.

Bates, M. J. (2005). An introduction to metatheories, theories, and models. In K. E. Fisher, S. Erdelez & L. McKechnie (Eds.), *Theories of information behavior* (pp. 1–24). Medford, NJ: Information Today.

Bates, M. J. (2006). Fundamental forms of information. *Journal of the American Society for Information Science and Technology, 57,* 1033–1045.

Bateson, G. (1972). *Steps to an ecology of mind.* New York: Ballantine Books.

Bauer, R. A. (1972). The obstinate audience: The influence process from the point of view of social communication. In W. Schramm & D. F. Roberts (Eds.), *The process and effects of mass communication* (pp. 326–346). Urbana: University of Illinois Press.

Becker, G. S., & Murphy, K. M. (1992). The division of labor, coordination costs, and knowledge. *Quarterly Journal of Economics, 107* (4), 1137–1160.

Becker, M. H., Maiman, L. A., Kirsch, J. P., Haefner, D. P., & Drachman, R. H. (1977). The Health Belief Model and prediction of dietary compliance: A field experiment. *Journal of Health and Social Behavior, 18,* 348–366.

Becker, M. H., & Rosenstock, I. M. (1989). Health promotion, disease prevention, and program retention. In H. E. Freeman & S. Levine (Eds.), *Handbook of medical sociology* (pp. 284–305). Inglewood Cliffs, NJ: Prentice Hall.

Becker, M. H., & Rosenstock, I. M. (1984). Compliance with medical advice. In A. Steptoe & A. Mathews (Eds.), *Health Care and Human Behavior* (pp. 175–208). London: Academic Press.

Bell, J. (1998). The new genetics in clinical practice. *British Medical Journal, 316,* 618–620.

Benson, J. K. (1975). The interorganizational network as a political economy. *Administrative Science Quarterly, 20,* 229–249.

Berelson, B. R., Lazarsfeld, P. F., & McPhee, W. N. (1954). *Voting: A study of opinion formation in a presidential campaign.* Chicago: University of Chicago Press.

Berger, C. R. (2011). From explanation to application. *Journal of Applied Communication Research, 39* (2), 214–222. doi: 10.1080/00909882.2011.556141.

Berlo, D. K. (1960). *The process of communication: An introduction to theory and practice.* New York: Holt, Rinehart and Winston.

Bettinghaus, E. P. (1986). Health promotion and the knowledge-attitude-behavior continuum. *Preventive Medicine, 15,* 475–491.

Bilodeau, B. A., & Degner, L. F. (1996). Information needs, sources of information, and decisional roles in women with breast cancer. *Oncology Nursing Forum, 23,* 691–696.

Black, M. (1979). More about metaphor. In A. Ortony (Ed.), *Metaphor and thought* (pp. 19–43). Cambridge: Cambridge University Press.

Bluman, L. G., Rimer, B. K., Berry, D. A., Borstelmann, N., Iglehart, J. D., Regan, K., . . . Winer, E. P. (1999). Attitudes, knowledge, and risk perceptions of women with breast and/or ovarian cancer considering testing for BRCA1 and BRCA2. *Journal of Clinical Oncology, 17,* 1040–1046.

Blumenthal, D. (2010). Expecting the unexpected: Health information technology and medical professionalism. In D. J. Rothman (Ed.), *Medical professionalism in the new information age* (pp. 8–22). New Brunswick, NJ: Rutgers University Press.

Bochner, A. P. (1982). On the efficacy of openness in close relationships. In M. Burgoon (Ed.), *Communication yearbook 5* (pp. 109–144). New Brunswick, NJ: Transaction Books.

Bochner, A. P. (1984). The functions of human communicating in interpersonal bonding. In C. C. Arnold & J. W. Bower (Eds.), *Handbook of rhetorical and communication theory* (pp. 554–621). Boston: Allyn and Bacon.

Borisoff, D., & Hahn, D. F. (1993). Thinking with the body: Sexual metaphors. *Communication Quarterly, 41* (3), 253–260.

Bottorff, J. L., Ratner, P. A., Johnson, J. L., Lovato, C. Y., & Joab, S. A. (1998). Communicating cancer risk information: The challenges of uncertainty. *Patient Education and Counseling, 33,* 67–81.

Boulos, M. N. K., & Wheeler, S. (2007). The emerging Web 2.0 social software: An enabling suite of sociable technologies in health and health care education. *Health Information and Library Journals, 24,* 2–23.

Boxenbaum, E., & Rouleau, L. (2011). New knowledge products as a bricolage: Metaphors and scripts in organizational theory. *Academy of Management Review, 36* (2), 272–296.

Bradley, E. H., Webster, T. R., Baker, D., Schlesinger, M., Inouye, S. K., Barth, M. C., . . . Koren, M. J. (2004). Translating research into practice: Speeding the adoption of innovative health care programs. The Commonwealth Fund. Retrieved from http://www.commonwealthfund.org/publications/publications_show. htm?doc_id=233248.

Brashers, D. E., Goldsmith, D. J., & Hsieh, E. (2002). Information seeking and avoiding in health contexts. *Human Communication Research, 28*, 258–272.

Brashers, D. E., Neidig, J. L., Haas, S. M., Dobbs, L. K., Cardillo, L. W., & Russell, J. A. (2000). Communication and the management of uncertainty: The case of persons living with HIV or AIDS. *Communication Monographs, 67*, 63–84.

Breiger, R. 1. (2004). The analysis of social networks. In M. Hardy & A. Bryman (Eds.), *Handbook of data analysis* (pp. 505–526). Thousand Oaks, CA: Sage.

Bronstein, L. R. (2003). A model for interdisciplinary collaboration. *Social Work, 48* (3), 297–306.

Brown, J. B., Stewart, M., & Ryan, B. L. (2003). Outcomes of patient-provider interaction. In T. L. Thompson, A. M. Dorsey, K. I. Miller & R. Parrott (Eds.), *Handbook of health communication* (pp. 141–161). Mahwah, NJ: Lawrence Erlbaum Associates.

Brown, J. S., & Duguid, P. (2002). *The social life of information*. Boston: Harvard Business School Press.

Buller, D. B., Borland, R., Woodall, W. G., Hall, J. R., Hines, J. M., Burris-Woodall, P., . . . Saba, L. (2008). Randomized trials on Consider This, a tailored, Internet-delivered smoking prevention program for adolescents. *Health Education and Behavior, 35* (2), 260–281. doi: 10.1177/1090198106288982.

Bunn, J., Bosompra, K., Ashikaga, T., Flynn, B., & Worden, J. (2002). Factors influencing intention to obtain a genetic test for colon cancer risk: A population-based study. *Preventive Medicine, 34*, 567–577.

Burt, R. S. (1987). Social contagion and innovation: Cohesion versus structural equivalence. *American Journal of Sociology, 92*, 1287–1335.

Burt, R. S. (1992). *Structural holes: The social structure of competition*. Cambridge, MA: Harvard University Press.

Burt, R. S. (2000). The network structure of social capital. *Research in Organization Behavior, 22*, 345–423.

Burt, R. S. (2002). Bridge decay. *Social Networks, 24*, 333–363.

Burt, R. S. (2004). Structural holes and good ideas. *American Journal of Sociology, 110*, 349–399.

Burt, R. S. (2005). *Brokerage and closure: An introduction to social capital*. New York: Oxford University Press.

Burt, R. S. (2007). Secondhand brokerage: Evidence on the importance of local structure for managers, bankers, and analysts. *Academy of Management Journal, 50*, 119–148.

Calnan, M. W. (1984). The Health Belief Model and participation in programmes for the early detection of breast cancer: A comparative analysis. *Social Science and Medicine, 19*, 823–830.

Cameron, A. F., & Webster, J. (2005). Unintended consequences of emerging communication technologies: Instant messaging in the workplace. *Computers in Human Behavior, 21*, 85–103. doi: 10.1016/j.chb.2003.12.001.

Carley, K. (1986). An approach for relating social structure to cognitive structure. *Journal of Mathematical Sociology, 12*, 137–189.

Case, D., Johnson, J. D., Andrews, J. E., Allard, S., & Kelly, K. M. (2004). From two-step flow to the Internet: The changing array of sources for genetics information seeking. *Journal of the American Society for Information Science and Technology, 55,* 660–669.

Case, D. O. (2008). Collection of family health histories: The link between genealogy and public health. *Journal of the American Society for Information Science and Technology, 59* (14), 2312–2319. doi: 10.1002/asi.20938.

Case, D. O. (2012). *Looking for information* (3rd ed.). Bingley, UK: Emerald Group Publishing.

Case, D. O., Andrews, J. E., Johnson, J. D., & Allard, S. L. (2005). Avoiding versus seeking: The relationship of information seeking to avoidance, blunting, coping, dissonance and related concepts. *Journal of Medical Libraries Association, 93,* 48–57.

Chaffee, S. H. (1979). *Mass media vs. interpersonal channels: The synthetic competition.* Paper presented at the Annual Convention of the Speech Communication Association, San Antonio, TX.

Champion, V. L. (1985). Use of the Health Belief Model in determining frequency of breast self-examination. *Research in Nursing and Health, 8,* 373–379.

Champion, V. L. (1987). The relationship of breast self-examination to Health Belief Model variables. *Research in Nursing and Health, 10,* 375–382.

Chen, C., & Hernon, P. (1982). *Information seeking: Assessing and anticipating user needs.* New York: Neal-Schuman Publishers.

Cheney, G., & Ashcraft, K. L. (2007). Considering "the professional" in communication studies: Implications for theory and research within and beyond the boundaries of organizational communication. *Communication Theory, 17,* 146–175.

Choi, B. C. K. (2005). Understanding the basic principles of knowledge translation. *Journal of Epidemiological Community Health, 59,* 93.

Cialdini, R. B. (2001). *Influence: Science and practice* (4th ed.). Boston: Allyn and Bacon.

Clark, P. G. (2006). What would a theory of interprofessional education look like? Some suggestions for developing a theoretical framework for team work training. *Journal of Interprofessional Care, 20,* 577–589.

Clarke, J. N., & Everest, M. (2006). Cancer in the mass print media: Fear, uncertainty and the medical model. *Social Science and Medicine 62* (10), 2591–2600.

Cloud, J. (2009, November 9). How a sugar pill can heal (or hurt). *Time,* 59.

Cloven, D. H., & Roloff, M. E. (1991). Sense-making activities and interpersonal conflict: Communicative cures for the mulling blues. *Western Journal of Speech Communication, 55* (Spring), 134–158.

Coberly, E., Boren, S. A., Davis, J. W., McConnell, A. L., Chitima-Matsiga, R., Ge, B., . . . Hodge, R. H. (2010). Linking clinic patients to Internet-based, condition-specific information prescriptions. *Journal of the Medical Library Association, 98* (2), 160–164.

Cohen, M. D., & March, J. G. (1986). *Leadership and ambiguity: The American college president* (2nd ed.). Boston: Harvard Business School.

Coiera, E. (2003). *Guide to health informatics* (2nd ed.). London: Arnold.

Cole, C., & Leide, J. E. (2006). A cognitive framework for human information behavior: The place of metaphor in human information organizing behavior. In A. Spink & C. Cole (Eds.), *New direction in human information behavior* (pp. 171–202). Rotterdam, Netherlands: Springer.

Cole, R. E., & Wagner, D. W. (1990). The pros and cons of the mass media colorectal screening program. In P. F. Engstrom, B. Rimer & L. E. Mortensen (Eds.), *Advances in cancer control: Screening and prevention research* (pp. 325–330). New York: Wiley.

Coleman, J., Katz, E., & Menzel, H. (1957). The diffusion of an innovation among physicians. *Sociometry, 20,* 253–270.

Colineau, N., & Paris, C. (2010). Talking about your health to strangers: Understanding the use of online social networks by patients. *New Review of Hypermedia and Multimedia, 16* (1–2), 141–160. doi: 10.1080/13614568.2010.496131.

Collins, F. S., Green, E. D., Guttmacher, A. E., & Guyer, M. S. (2003). A vision for the future of genomics research: A blueprint for the genomic era. *Nature, 422,* 1–13.

Collins, F. S., & McKusick, V. A. (2001). Implications of the Human Genome Project for medical science. *Journal of the American Medical Association, 285* (5), 540–544.

Collins, R. (1981). On the microfoundations of macrosociology. *American Journal of Sociology, 86,* 984–1014.

Condit, C. M. (1999). *The meanings of the gene: Public debates about human heredity.* Madison: University of Wisconsin Press.

Cornelissen, J. P. (2005). Beyond compare: Metaphor in organization theory. *Academy of Management Review, 30,* 751–764.

Cornelissen, J. P. (2006). Metaphor in organization theory: Progress and the past. *Academy of Management Review, 31,* 485–488.

Cotten, S. R., & Gupta, S. S. (2004). Characteristics of online and offline health information seekers and factors that discriminate between them. *Social Science and Medicine, 59,* 1795–1806. doi: 10.1016/j.socscimed.2004.02.020.

Crawford, E. B., & Lepine, J. A. (2013). A configural theory of team processes: Accounting for the structure of taskwork and teamwork. *Academy of Management Review, 38* (1), 32–48.

Crespo, J. (2004). Training the health information seeker: Quality issues in health information Web sites. *Library Trends, 53* (2), 360–374.

Cross, R., Rice, R. E., & Parker, A. (2001). Information seeking in social context: Structural influences and receipt of information benefits. *IEEE Transactions on Systems, Man, and Cybernetics—Part C: Applications and Reviews, 31,* 438–448.

Croyle, R. T., & Lerman, C. (1999). Risk communication in genetic testing for cancer susceptibility. *Journal of National Cancer Institute, 25,* 59–66.

Cullen, P., Cottingham, P., Doolan, J., Edgar, B., Ellis, C., Fisher, M., . . . Whittington, J. (2001). Knowledge seeking strategies of natural resource professionals (Technical Report 2/2001 ed.) Canberra, Australia: Cooperative Research Centre for Freshwater Ecology.

Cullen, P. W., Norris, R. H., Resh, V. H., Reynoldson, T. B., Rosenberg, D. M., & Barbour, M. T. (1999). Collaboration in scientific research: A critical need for freshwater ecology. *Freshwater Biology, 42*, 131–142.

Cummings, K. M., Becker, M. H., & Maile, M. C. (1980). Bringing the models together: An empirical approach to combining variables used to explain health actions. *Journal of Behavioral Medicine, 3*, 123–145.

D'Amour, D., Ferrada-Videla, M., Rodriguez, L. S. M., & Beaulieu, M. D. (2005). The conceptual basis for interprofessional collaboration: Core concepts and theoretical frameworks. *Journal of Interprofessional Care, Supplement 1*, 116–131.

Dai, Q., & Kauffman, R. J. (2002). B2B e-commerce revisited: Leading perspectives on the key issues and research directions. *Electronic Markets, 12*, 67–83.

Dance, F. E. X. (1970). The "concept" of communication. *Journal of Communication, 20*, 201–210.

Danes, J. E., Hunter, J. E., & Woelfel, J. (1978). Mass communication and belief change: A test of three mathematical models. *Human Communication Research, 4*, 243–252.

Davenport, T. H., & Prusak, L. (1998). *Working knowledge: How organizations manage what they know.* Boston: Harvard Business School Press.

Dawson, E., Savitsky, K., & Dunning, D. (2006). "Don't tell me. I don't want to know": Understanding people's reluctance to obtain medical diagnostic information. *Journal of Applied Social Psychology, 36* (3), 751–768.

Deal, T., & Kennedy, A. (1982). *Corporate cultures.* Reading, MA: Addison-Wesley.

Dearing, J. (May 2000). Dilemmas of evaluation research. *ICA News, 5* & 7.

Dearing, J. W. (2006). *The emerging science of translational research.* Paper presented at the Kentucky Conference on Health Communication, Lexington, KY.

Dearing, J. W., & Kreuter, M. W. (2010). Designing for diffusion: How can we increase uptake of cancer communication innovations? *Patient Education and Counseling, 81S*, S100–S110. doi: 10.1016/j.pec.2010.10.013.

Dearing, J. W., Meyer, G., & Kazmierczak, J. (1994). Portraying the new: Communication between university innovators and potential users. *Science Communication, 16*, 11–42.

Degner, L. F., & Sloan, J. A. (1992). Decision-making during serious illness: What role do patients really want to play? *Journal of Clinical Psychology, 45*, 941–950.

Dervin, B. (1980). Communication gaps and inequities: Moving toward a reconceptualization. In B. Dervin & M. J. Voight (Eds.), *Progress in communication sciences* (pp. 74–112). Norwood, NJ: ABLEX.

Dervin, B. (1989). Users as research inventions: How research categories perpetuate inequities. *Journal of Communication, 39*, 216–232.

DiClemente, C. C., & Prochaska, J. O. (1985). Processes and stages of self-change: Coping and competence in smoking behavior change. In S. Shiffman & T. A. Wills (Eds.), *Coping and substance use* (pp. 319–343). New York: Academic Press.

Dijkstra, M., Buijtels, H. J. J. M., & VanRaaij, W. F. (2005). Separate and joint effects of medium type on consumer responses: A comparison of television, print, and the Internet. *Journal of Business Research, 58*, 377–386.

Dillard, J. P. (1994). Rethinking the study of fear appeals. *Communication Theory 4*, 295–323.

Dobos, J. (1988). Choices of new media and traditional channels in organizations. *Communication Research Reports, 5*, 131–139.

Dockterman, E. (2012, November 12). Playing for keeps. Smart-phone games could make healthy care more fun-effective. *Time.* www.time.com/time/magazine/article/0,9171,2128297,00.html.

Doctor, R. D. (1992). Social equity and information technologies: Moving toward information democracy. In M. E. Williams (Ed.), *Annual review of information science and technology* (pp. 44–96). Medford, NJ: Learned Information.

Donohew, L., Helm, D. M., Cook, P. L., & Shatzer, M. J. (1987). *Sensation seeking, marijuana use, and responses to prevention campaigns.* Paper presented at the International Communication Association, Montreal.

Donohew, L., Palmgreen, P., Zimmerman, R., Harrington, N., & Lane, D. (2003). Health risk takers and prevention. In D. Romer (Ed.), *Reducing adolescent risk: Toward an integrated approach* (pp. 165–170). Thousand Oaks, CA: Sage.

Dorsey, A. M. (2003). Lessons and challenges from the field. In T. L. Thompson, A. M. Dorsey, K. I. Miller & R. Parrott (Eds.), *Handbook of health communication* (pp. 607–608). Mahwah, NJ: Lawrence Erlbaum.

Dorsey, A. M., Scherer, C. W., & Real, K. (1999). The college tradition of "drink 'til you drop": The relation between students' social networks and engaging in risky behaviors. *Health Communication, 11* (4), 313–334.

Downs, A. (1967). *Inside bureaucracy.* Boston: Little, Brown.

Drazin, R., Glynn, M. A., & Kazanjian, R. K. (1999). Multilevel theorizing about creativity in organizations: A sensemaking perspective. *Academy of Management Review, 24*, 296–307.

Drucker, P. F. (1974). *Management—tasks, responsibilities, practices.* New York: Harper and Row.

Duggan, A. P., & Thompson, T. L. (2011). Provider-patient interaction and related outcomes. In T. L. Thompson, R. Parrott & J. F. Nussbaum (Eds.), *The Routledge handbook of health communication* (pp. 414–427). New York: Routledge.

Durfy, S. J., Bowen, D. J., McTiernan, A., Sporleder, J., & Burke, W. (1999). Attitudes and interest in genetic testing for breast and ovarian cancer susceptibility in diverse groups of women in western Washington. *Cancer Epidemiology, Biomarkers and Prevention, 8*, 369–375.

Edgar, T., Volkman, J. E., & Logan, A. M. B. (2011). Social marketing: Its meaning, use, and application for health. In T. L. Thompson, R. Parrott & J. F. Nussbaum (Eds.), *The Routledge handbook of health communication* (2nd ed., pp. 235–251). New York: Routledge.

Edmondson, A. C., Bohmer, R. M., & Pisano, G. P. (2001). Disrupted routines: Team learning and new technology implementation in hospitals. *Administrative Science Quarterly, 46*, 685–716.

Eggert, L. L., & Parks, M. R. (1987). Communication network involvement in adolescent's friendships and romantic relationships. In M. L. McLaughlin (Ed.), *Communication yearbook 10* (pp. 283–322). Beverly Hills, CA: Sage.

Eisenberg, E. M., Contractor, N. S., & Monge, P. R. (1988). *Semantic networks in organizations.* Paper presented at the International Communication Association, New Orleans, LA.

Elliott, D. S., & Mihalic, S. (2004). Issues in disseminating and replicating effective prevention programs. *Prevention Science, 5,* 47–53.

Entman, R. M., & Wildman, S. S. (1992). Reconciling economic and noneconomic perspectives on media policy: Transcending the "marketplace of ideas." *Journal of Communication, 42,* 5–19.

Epstein, R. M., & Street, R. L., Jr. (2007). *Patient-centered communication in cancer care: Promoting healing and reducing suffering.* (NIH Publication No. 07-6225). Bethesda, MD: National Institutes of Health.

Eysenbach, G. (2005). Design and evaluation of consumer health information Web sites. In D. Lewis, G. Eysenbach, R. Kukafka, P. Z. Stavri & H. B. Jimison (Eds.), *Consumer health informatics: Informing consumers and improving health care* (pp. 34–60). New York: Springer.

Fan, D. P. (2002). Impact of persuasive information on secular trends and health-related behaviors. In R. C. Hornik (Ed.), *Public health communication: Evidence for behavior change* (pp. 251–264). Mahwah, NJ: Lawrence Erlbaum Associates.

Farace, R. V., Monge, P. R., & Russell, H. (1977). *Communicating and organizing.* Reading, MA: Addison-Wesley.

Farace, R. V., Taylor, J. A., & Stewart, J. P. (1978). Criteria for evaluation of organizational communication effectiveness: Review and synthesis. In D. Nimmo (Ed.), *Communication yearbook 2* (pp. 271–292). New Brunswick, NJ: Transaction Books.

Feldman, M. S., & March, J. G. (1981). Information in organizations as signal and symbol. *Administrative Science Quarterly, 26,* 171–186.

Ferguson, T. (2007). E-patients: How they can help us heal health care. E-patients. net. Retrieved from http://e-patients.net/e-Patients_White_Paper.pdf.

Fidler, L. A., & Johnson, J. D. (1984). Communication and innovation implementation. *Academy of Management Review, 9,* 704–711.

Firth-Cozens, J. (2004). Why communication fails in the operating room. *Quality and Safety in Health Care, 13,* 327. doi: 10.1136/qshc.2004.010785.

Fischoff, B. (1995). Risk perception and communication unplugged: Twenty years of process. *Risk Analysis, 15* (2), 137–145.

Fishbein, M., & Ajzen, I. (1975). *Beliefs, attitudes, intention, and behavior: An introduction to theory and research.* Reading, MA: Addisson-Wesley.

Fisher, W. R. (1987). *Human communication as narration: Toward a philosophy of reason, value, and action.* Columbia: University of South Carolina Press.

Flay, B. R. (1987). Mass media and smoking cessation: A critical review. *American Journal of Public Health, 77,* 153–160.

Flay, B. R., DiTecco, D., & Schlegel, R. P. (1980). Mass media in health promotion: An analysis using an extended information processing model. *Health Education Quarterly, 7,* 127–147.

Flora, J. A., Maccoby, N., & Farquhar, J. W. (1989). Communication campaigns to prevent cardiovascular disease: The Stanford Community Studies. In R. E. Rice

& C. K. Atkin (Eds.), *Public communication campaigns* (2nd ed., pp. 233–252). Newbury Park, CA: Sage.

Fonner, K. L., & Roloff, M. E. (2010). Why teleworkers are more satisfied with their jobs than are office-based workers: When less contact is beneficial. *Journal of Applied Communication Research, 38* (4), 336–361. doi: 10.1080/00909882.2010.513998.

Fonner, K. L., & Roloff, M. E. (2012). Testing the connectivity paradox: Linking teleworkers' communication media use to social presence, stress from interruptions, and organizational identification. *Communication Monographs, 29* (2), 203–231. doi: 10.1080/0367751.2012.673000.

Fontaine, M. A. (2004). Keeping communities of practice afloat: Understanding and fostering roles in communities. In E. Lesser & L. Prusak (Eds.), *Creating value with knowledge: Insights from the IBM Institute for Business Value* (pp. 124–133). New York: Oxford University Press.

Ford, E. W., Duncan, J. W., Bedeian, A. G., Ginter, P. M., Rousculp, M. D., & Adams, A. M. (2003). Mitigating risks, visible hands, inevitable disasters, and soft variables. *Academy of Management Executive, 17,* 46–60.

Ford, L. A., Babrow, A. S., & Stohl, C. (1996). Social support messages and the management of uncertainty in the experience of breast cancer: An application of problematic integration theory. *Commuication Monographs, 63,* 189–207.

Form, W. H. (1972). Technology and social behavior of workers in four countries: A sociotechnical perspective. *American Sociological Review, 37,* 727–738.

Fortner, R. S. (1995). Excommunication in the information society. *Critical Studies in Mass Communication, 12,* 133–154.

Fox, S., & Jones, S. (2009, June 11). The social life of health information. Pew Internet. Retrieved from http://www.pewinternet.org/Reports/2009/8-The-Social-Life-of-Health-Information.aspx.

Freeman, A. C., & Sweeney, K. (2001). Why general practitioners do not implement evidence: Qualitative study. *British Medical Journal, 323,* 1100–1110.

Freimuth, V. S. (1987). The diffusion of supportive information. In T. L. Albrecht & M. B. Adelman (Eds.), *Communicating social support* (pp. 212–237). Newbury Park, CA: Sage.

Freimuth, V. S. (1990). The chronically uninformed: Closing the knowledge gap in health. In E. B. Ray & L. Donohew (Eds.), *Communication and health: Systems and applications* (pp. 171–186). Hillsdale, NJ: Lawrence Erlbaum Associates.

Freimuth, V. S., Stein, J. A., & Kean, T. J. (1989). *Searching for health information: The Cancer Information Service model.* Philadelphia: University of Pennsylvania Press.

French, J. R. P. (1956). A formal theory of social power. *Psychological Review, 63,* 181–194.

French, J. R. P., Jr., & Raven, B. (1959). The bases of social power. In D. Cartwright (Ed.), *Studies in social power* (pp. 150–167). Ann Arbor, MI: Institute for Social Research.

Frost, P. J. (1987). Power, politics, and influence. In F. M. Jablin, L. L. Putnam, K. H. Roberts & L. W. Porter (Eds.), *Handbook of organizational communication: An interdisciplinary perspective* (pp. 503–548). Newbury Park, CA: Sage.

Fund for the Improvement of Postsecondary Education (FIPSE). (2003). *Innovation and impact: The comprehensive program FY 2004.* Washington, DC: FIPSE.

Galbraith, J. R. (1982). Designing the innovating organization. *Organizational Dynamics, 10,* 5–25.

Garg, A. X., Adhikari, N. K. J., McDonald, H., Rosas-Arellano, M. P., Devereaux, P. J., Beyene, J., . . . Haynes, R. B. (2005). Effects of computerized clinical decision support systems on practitioner performance and patient outcomes. *Journal of American Medical Association, 293,* 1223–1238.

Gargiulo, M., & Benassi, M. (2000). Trapped in your own net? Network cohesion, structural holes, and the adaption of social capital. *Organization Science, 11,* 183–196.

Garrett, R. K. (2009). Politically motivated reinforcement seeking: Reframing the selective exposure debate. *Journal of Communication, 59,* 676–699.

Geertz, C. (1973). *The interpretation of cultures.* New York: Basic Books.

Geertz, C. (1978). The bazaar economy: Information and search in peasant marketing. *American Economic Review, 68,* 28–37.

Geller, G., Berhnhardt, B. A., Helzlsouer, K., Holtzman, N. A., Stefanek, M., & Wilcox, P. M. (1995). Informed consent and BRCA1 testing. *Nature Genetics, 11,* 364.

Gillotti, C. M. (2003). Medical disclosure and decision-making: Excavating the complexities of physician-patient information exchange. In T. L. Thompson, A. M. Dorsey, K. I. Miller & R. Parrott (Eds.), *Handbook of health communication* (pp. 163–181). Mahwah, NJ: Lawrence Erlbaum Associates.

Given, B. A., Given, C. W., & Kozachik, S. (2001). Family support in advanced cancer. *CA Cancer Journal for Clinicians, 51* (4), 213–231.

Glasgow, R. E., Klesges, L. M., Dzewaltowski, D. A., Bull, S. S., & Estabrooks, P. (2004). The future of health behavior change research: What is needed to improve translation of research into health promotion practice. *Annals of Behavioral Medicine, 27,* 3–12.

Glasgow, R. E., Lichtenstein, E., & Marcus, A. C. (2003). Why don't we see more translation of health promotion research to practice? Rethinking the efficacy-to-effectiveness transition. *American Journal of Public Health, 93,* 1261–1267.

Glasgow, R. E., Marcus, A. G., Bull, S. S., & Wilson, K. M. (2004). Disseminating effective cancer screening interventions. *Cancer Supplement, 101,* 1239–1250. doi: 10.1002/cncr.20509.

Glasgow, R. E., Vogt, T. M., & Boles, S. M. (1999). Evaluating the public health impact of health promotion interventions: The RE-AIM framework. *American Journal of Public Health, 89,* 1322–1327.

Gleick, J. (2011). *The information: A history, a theory, a flood.* New York: Pantheon Books.

Goffman, E. (1974). *Frame analysis: An essay on the organization of experience.* Cambridge, MA: Harvard University Press.

Goldberg, S. C. (1954). Three situational determinants of conformity to social norms. *Journal of Abnormal and Social Psychology, 9,* 449–459.

Goldsmith, D. (2001). A normative approach to the study of uncertainty and communication. *Journal of Communication, 51* (3), 514–533.

Goldsmith, D. J., & Albrecht, T. L. (2011). Social support, social networks, and health: A guiding framework. In T. L. Thompson, R. Parrott & J. F. Nussbaum (Eds.), *The Routledge handbook of health communication* (pp. 335–348). New York: Routledge.

Goodall, H. L. (1989). On becoming an organizational detective: The role of context, sensitivity, and intuitive logics in communication consulting. *Southern Communication Journal, 55*, 42–54.

Gouran, D. S., & Hirokawa, R. Y. (2003). Effective decision making and problem solving in groups: A functional perspective. In R. Y. Hirokawa, R. S. Cathcart, L. A. Samovar & L. D. Henman (Eds.), *Small group communication: Theory and practice* (pp. 27–38). New York: Oxford University Press.

Govindarajan, V., & Trimble, C. (2005). Organizational DNA for strategic innovation. *California Management Review, 47*, 47–76.

Granovetter, M. S. (1982). The strength of weak ties: A network theory revisited. In P. V. Marsden & N. Lin (Eds.), *Social structure in network analysis* (pp. 105–130). Beverly Hills, CA: Sage.

Grant, D., & Oswick, C. (1996). Introduction: Getting the measure of metaphors. In D. Grant & C. Oswick (Eds.), *Metaphor and organizations* (pp. 1–20). Thousand Oaks, CA: Sage.

Gray, B. (1996). Review of *Frame reflection. Academy of Management Review, 21*, 576–579.

Gray, S. W., O'Grady, C., Karp, L., Smith, D., Schwartz, J. S., Hornik, R. C., & Armstrong, K. (2009). Risk information exposure and direct-to-consumer genetic testing for BRCA mutations among women with a personal or family history of breast or ovarian cancer. *Cancer Epidemiology, Biomarkers, and Prevention, 18* (4), 1303–1311.

Green, L. A., & Seifert, C. M. (2005). Translation of research into practice: Why we can't "just do it." *JABFP, 18*, 541–545.

Green, L. W., & Glasgow, R. E. (2006). Evaluating the relevance, generalization, and applicability of research: Issues in external validation and translation methodology. *Evaluation and the Health Professions, 29*, 126–153.

Gregory, K. L. (1983). Native-view paradigms: Multiple cultures and culture conflicts in organizations. *Administrative Science Quarterly, 28*, 359–376.

Grimshaw, J. M., Thomas, R. E., MacLennan, G., Fraser, C., Ramsay, C. R., Vale, L., . . . Donaldson, C. (2004). Effectiveness and efficiency of guideline dissemination and implementation strategies. *Health Technology Assessment, 8*, viii–73.

Grol, R. (2002). Changing physicians' competence and performance: Finding the balance between the individual and the organization. *Journal of Continuing Education in the Health Professions, 22*, 244–251.

Grol, R., & Grimshaw, J. (2003). From best evidence to best practice: Effective implementation change in patients' care. *Lancet, 362*, 1225–1230.

Groopman, J. (2007). *How doctors think.* New York: Houghton Mifflin.

Gulati, R. (2007). *Managing network resources: Alliances, affiliations, and other relational assets.* New York: Oxford University Press.

Gustafson, D. H., Hawkins, R., McTavish, F., Pingree, S., Chen, W. C., Volrathongchai, K., . . . Serlin, R. C. (2008). Internet-based interactive support for cancer patients: Are integrated systems better? *Journal of Communication, 58*, 238–257.

Guttman, N. (2011). Ethics in communication for health promotion in clinical settings and campaigns. In T. L. Thompson, R. Parrott & J. F. Nussbaum (Eds.), *The Routledge handbook of health communication* (pp. 632–636). New York: Routledge.

Hall, H. J. (1981). Patterns in the use of information: The right to be different. *Journal of American Society for Information Science, 32*, 103–112.

Hanneman, G. J. (1973). Communicating drug-abuse information among college students. *Public Opinion Quarterly, 37*, 171–197.

Hansen, M. T. (1999). The search-transfer problem: The role of weak ties in sharing knowledge across organization subunits. *Administrative Science Quarterly, 44*, 82–111.

Hansen, M. T., & Haas, M. R. (2001). Competing for attention in knowledge markets: Electronic document dissemination in a management consulting company. *Administrative Science Quarterly, 46*, 1–28.

Haskard, K. B., Williams, S. L., & DiMatteo, M. R. (2009). Physician-patient communication: Psychosocial care, emotional well-being, and health outcomes. In D. E. Brashers & D. J. Goldsmith (Eds.), *Communicating to manage health and illness* (pp. 15–40). New York: Routledge.

Health and Human Services. (2010). *National Action Plan to Improve Health Literacy*. Retrieved from: http://www.health.gov/communication/HLActionPlan/pdf/Health_Lit_Action_Plan_Summary.pdf.

Helmes, A. W., Bowen, D. J., Bowden, R., & Bengel, J. (2000). Predictors of participation in genetic research in a primary case physician network. *Cancer Epidemiology, Biomarkers, and Prevention, 9*, 1377–1379.

Hesse, B. W., Johnson, L. E., & Davis, K. L. (2010). Extending the reach, effectiveness, and efficiency of communication: Evidence from the centers of excellence in cancer communication research. *Patient Education and Counseling, 81S*, S1–S5. doi: 10.1016/j.pec.2010.11.002.

Hibbard, J. H. (2003). Engaging health care consumers to improve the quality of care. *Medical Care, 41*, I-60–I-70.

Hickson, D. J. (1987). Decision making at the top of organizations. *Annual Review of Sociology, 13*, 165–192.

Hill, D., Gardner, G., & Rassaby, J. (1985). Factors predisposing women to take precautions against breast and cervix cancer. *Journal of Applied Social Psychology, 15*, 59–79.

Hinds, P. J., & Pfeffer, J. (2003). Why organizations don't "know what they know": Cognitive and motivational factors affecting the transfer of expertise. In M. S. Ackerman, V. Pipek & V. Wulf (Eds.), *Sharing expertise: Beyond knowledge management* (pp. 3–26). Cambridge, MA: MIT Press.

Hines, S. C. (2001). Coping with uncertainties in advance care planning. *Journal of Communication, 51* (3), 498–513.

Hirokawa, R. Y. (1996). Communication and group decision making efficacy. In R. S. Cathcart, L. A. Samovar & L. D. Henman (Eds.), *Small group communication: Theory and practice*. Madison, WI: Brown and Benchmark.

Hirokawa, R. Y., DeGooyer, D. H., Jr., & Valde, K. S. (2003). *Characteristics of effective health care teams*. Oxford, UK: Roxbury Publishing Co.

Hjorland, B. (2007). Information: Objective or subjective/situational? *Journal of the American Society for Information Science and Technology, 58,* 1448–1456.

Hoffman, G. M. (1994). *The technology payoff: How to profit with empowered workers in the information age.* New York: Irwin.

Holmes, M. E. (1994). *An alternative root metaphor for small group communication research.* Paper presented at the Speech Communication Association, New Orleans, Lousiana.

Hornik, R. C. (2002a). Epilogue: Evaluation design for public health communication programs. In R. C. Hornik (Ed.), *Public health communication: Evidence for behavior change* (pp. 385–405). Mahwah, NJ: Lawrence Erlbaum Associates.

Hornik, R. C. (2002b). Introduction, public health communication: Making sense of contradictory evidence. In R. C. Hornik (Ed.), *Public health communication: Evidence for behavior change* (pp. 1–19). Mahwah, NJ: Lawrence Erlbaum Associates.

Huckfeldt, R., Johnson, P. E., & Sprague, J. (2004). *Political disagreement: The survival of diverse opinions within communication networks.* New York: Cambridge University Press.

Hurley, R. J., Kosenko, K. A., & Brashers, D. (2011). Uncertain terms: Message features of online cancer news. *Communication Monographs, 78* (3), 370–390. doi: 10.1080/03637751.2011.565061.

Hutchings, D. (1998). Communicating with metaphor: A dance with many veils. *American Journal of Hospice and Palliative Medicine, 15,* 282–284. doi: 10.1177/104990919801500510.

Huysman, M., & van Baalen, P. (2002). Editorial. *Trends in Communication, 8,* 3–5.

Jallinoja, P., Hakonen, A., Aro, A. R., Niemela, P., Hietala, M., Lonnqvist, J., . . . Aula, P. (1998). Attitudes towards genetic testing: Analysis of contradictions. *Social science medicine C, 46,* 1367–1374.

Janis, I., & Feshback, S. (1953). Effects of fear-arousing communications. *Journal of Abnormal and Social Psychology, 48,* 78–92.

Janz, N. H., & Becker, M. H. (1984). The Health Belief Model: A decade later. *Health Education Quarterly, 11,* 1–47.

Johnson, B., & Hagstrom, B. (2005). The translation perspective as an alternate to the policy diffusion paradigm: The case of the Swedish methadone maintenance treatment. *Journal of Social Policy, 34,* 365–389.

Johnson, J. D. (1983). A test of a model of magazine exposure and appraisal in India. *Communication Monographs, 50,* 148–157.

Johnson, J. D. (1984a). International communication media appraisal: Tests in Germany. In R. N. Bostrom (Ed.), *Communication yearbook 8* (pp. 645–658). Beverly Hills, CA: Sage.

Johnson, J. D. (1984b). Media exposure and appraisal: Phase II, tests of a model in Nigeria. *Journal of Applied Communication Research, 12,* 63–74.

Johnson, J. D. (1987). A model of international communication media appraisal: Phase IV, generalizing the model to film. *International Journal of Intercultural Relations, 11,* 129–142.

Johnson, J. D. (1990). Effects of communicative factors on participation in innovations. *Journal of Business Communication, 27,* 7–24.

Johnson, J. D. (1993a). *Organizational communication structure*. Norwood, NJ: ABLEX.

Johnson, J. D. (1993b). *Tests of a comprehensive model of cancer-related information seeking*. Paper presented at the Speech Communication Association, Miami, FL.

Johnson, J. D. (1997a). *Cancer-related information seeking*. Cresskill, NJ: Hampton Press.

Johnson, J. D. (1997b). A frameworks for interaction (FINT) scale: Extensions and refinement in an industrial setting. *Communication Studies, 48*, 127–141.

Johnson, J. D. (1998). Frameworks for interaction and disbandments: A case study. *Journal of Educational Thought, 32*, 5–21.

Johnson, J. D. (2003). On contexts of information seeking. *Information Processing and Management, 39*, 735–760.

Johnson, J. D. (2004). The emergence, maintenance, and dissolution of structural hole brokerage within consortia. *Communication Theory, 14*, 212–236.

Johnson, J. D. (2005). *Innovation and knowledge management: The Cancer Information Services Research Consortium*. Cheltenham, UK: Edward Elgar.

Johnson, J. D. (2009a). An impressionistic mapping of information behavior with special attention to contexts, rationality, and ignorance. *Information Processing and Management, 45*, 593–604.

Johnson, J. D. (2009b). Information regulation and work-life: Applying the Comprehensive Model of Information Seeking to organizational networks. In T. D. Afifi & W. A. Afifi (Eds.), *Uncertainty, information management, and disclosure decisions: Theories and applications* (pp. 182–199). New York: Routledge.

Johnson, J. D. (2009c). Profiling the likelihood of success of electronic medical records. In S. Kleinman (Ed.), *The culture of efficiency: Technology in everyday life* (pp. 121–141). New York: Peter Lang.

Johnson, J. D., Andrews, J., & Allard, S. (2001). A model for understanding and affecting cancer genetics information seeking. *Library and Information Science Research, 23*, 335–349.

Johnson, J. D., Andrews, J. E., Case, D. O., Allard, S. L., & Johnson, N. E. (2006). Fields and/or pathways: Contrasting and/or complementary views of information seeking. *Information Processing and Management, 42*, 569–582.

Johnson, J. D., & Case, D. O. (2012). *Health information seeking*. New York: Peter Lang.

Johnson, J. D., Donohue, W. A., Atkin, C. K., & Johnson, S. H. (1995). A comprehensive model of information seeking: Tests focusing on a technical organization. *Science Communication, 16*, 274–303.

Johnson, J. D., & Meischke, H. (1993a). Cancer-related channel selection: An extension for a sample of women who have had a mammogram. *Women and Health, 20*, 31–44.

Johnson, J. D., & Meischke, H. (1993b). A comprehensive model of cancer-related information seeking applied to magazines. *Human Communication Research, 19*, 343–367.

Johnson, J. D., & Oliveira, O. S. (1988). A model of international communication media appraisal and exposure: A comprehensive test in Belize. *World communication, 17*, 253–277.

Joshi, A. (2006). The influence of organizational demography on the external networking behavior of teams. *Academy of Management Journal, 31*, 583–595.

Kahneman, D., Slovic, P., & Tversky, A. (1982). *Judgment under uncertainty: Heuristics and biases.* New York: Cambridge University Press.

Kalman, M. E., Monge, P. R., Fulk, J., & Heino, R. (2002). Motivations to resolve communication dilemmas in database-mediated collaboration. *Communication Research, 29* (2), 125–154.

Kalyanaraman, S., & Sundar, S. S. (2008). Portrait of the portal as metaphor: Explicating Web portals for communication research. *Journalism and Mass Communication Quarterly, 85* (2), 239–256.

Kaplan, S. J. (1990). Visual metaphors in the representation of communication technology. *Critical Studies in Mass Communication, 7*, 37–47.

Kash, K. M., Ortega-Verdejo, K., Dabney, M. K., Holland, J. C., Miller, D. G., & Osborne, M. P. (2000). Psychosocial aspects of cancer genetics: Women at high risk for breast and ovarian cancer. *Seminars in Surgical Oncology, 18*, 333–338.

Katila, R., & Ahuja, G. (2002). Something old, something new: A longitudinal study of search behavior and new product introduction. *Academy of Management Journal, 45*, 1183–1194.

Katz, D., & Kahn, R. L. (1978). *The social psychology of organizations* (2nd ed.). New York: Wiley.

Katz, E. (1957). The two-step flow of communication: An up-to-date report on an hypothesis. *Public Opinion Quarterly, 21*, 61–78.

Katz, E. (1968). On reopening the question of selectivity in exposure to mass communications. In R. P. Abelson (Ed.), *Theories of cognitive consistency* (pp. 788–796). New York: Rand McNally.

Katz, E., Blumler, J. G., & Gurevitch, M. (1974). Uses of mass communication by the individual. In W. P. Davison (Ed.), *Mass communication research: Major issues and future directions* (pp. 11–35). New York: Praeger.

Katz, E., Gurevitch, M., & Haas, H. (1973). On the use of the mass media for important things. *American sociological review, 38*, 164–181.

Katz, E., & Lazersfeld, P. F. (1955). *Personal influence: The part played by people in the flow of mass communications.* New York: The Free Press.

Katz, N., Lazer, D., Arrow, H., & Contractor, N. (2004). Network theory and small groups. *Small Group Research, 35*, 307–332.

Keen, M., & Stocklmayer, S. (1999). Science communication: The evolving role of rural industry research and development corporations. *Australian Journal of Environmental Management, 6*, 196–206.

Kegeles, S. S. (1980). Review of the "Health Belief Model and personal health behavior." *Social science medicine C, 14*, 227–229.

Keller, R. T. (2001). Cross-functional product groups in research and new product development: Diversity, communications, job stress, and outcomes. *Academy of Management Journal, 44*, 547–555.

Kelly, K., Andrews, J. E., Case, D. O., Allard, S. L., & Johnson, J. D. (2007). Information seeking and intentions to have genetic testing for hereditary cancers in rural and Appalachian Kentuckians. *Journal of Rural Health, 23*, 166–172.

Kent, M. L. (2001). Managerial rhetoric as the metaphor for the World Wide Web. *Crtical Studies in Media Communication, 18* (3), 359–375.

Kilduff, M., & Tsai, W. (2003). *Social networks and organizations*. Thousand Oaks, CA: Sage.

Kilmann, R. H., Slevin, D. P., & Thomas, K. W. (1983). The problem of producing useful knowledge. In R. H. Kilmann, K. W. Thomas, D. P. Slevin, R. Nath & S. L. Jerrell (Eds.), *Producing useful knowledge for organizations* (pp. 1–21). San Francisco, CA: Jossey-Bass.

Kirman, A. (2001). Market organization and individual behavior: Evidence from fish markets. In J. E. Rauch & A. Casella (Eds.), *Networks and markets* (pp. 155–195). New York: Russell Sage.

Kirmeyer, S. L., & Lin, T. R. (1987). Social support: Its relationship to observed communication with peers and superiors. *Academy of Management Journal, 30*, 138–150.

Klausner, R. (1996). *The nation's investment in cancer research*. Bethesda, MD: National Cancer Institute.

Klein, G. (2009). *Streetlights and shadows: Searching for the keys to adaptive decision making*. Cambridge, MA: MIT Press.

Klesges, L. M., Estabrook, P. A., Dzewaltowski, D. A., Bull, S. S., & Glasgow, R. E. (2005). Beginning with application in mind: Designing and planning health behavior change interventions to enhance dissemination. *Annals of Behavioral Medicine, 29*, 66–75.

Koch, S., & Deetz, S. (1981). Metaphor analysis of social reality in organizations. *Journal of Applied Communication Research, 9* (1), 1–15.

Koop, C. E. (1995). Editorial: A personal role in health care reform. *American Journal of Public Health, 85*, 759–760.

Kratzer, J., Leenders, R. T. A. J., & van Engelen, J. M. L. (2004). Stimulating the potential: Creative performance and communication in innovation teams. *Creativity and Innovation Management, 13*, 63–71.

Kreps, G. L. (2009). Applying Weick's model of organizing to health care and health promotion: Highlighting the central role of health communication. *Patient Education and Counseling, 74*, 347–355. doi: 10.1016/j.pec.2008.12.002.

Krippendorf, K. (1986). *Information theory: Structural models for qualitative data*. Newbury Park, CA: Sage.

Krippendorf, K. (1993). Major metaphors of communication and some constructivist reflections on their use. *Cybernetics and Human Knowing, 2* (1), 3–25.

Kuhn, T. (2002). Negotiating boundaries between scholars and practitioners: Knowledge, networks, and communities of practice. *Management Communication Quarterly, 16*, 106–112.

Kukafka, R. (2005). Tailored health communication. In D. Lewis, G. Eysenbach, R. Kukafka, P. Z. Stavri & H. B. Jimison (Eds.), *Consumer health informatics: Informing consumers and improving health care* (pp. 22–33). New York: Springer.

Lakoff, G., & Johnson, M. (1980). *Metaphors we live by*. Chicago: University of Chicago Press.

Lammers, J. C., & Garcia, M. A. (2009). Exploring the concept of "profession" for organizational communication research. *Management Communication Quarterly, 22* (3), 357–381. doi: 10.1177/0893318908327007.

Lane, S. D. (1983). Compliance, satisfaction, and physician-patient communication. In R. N. Bostrom (Ed.), *Communication yearbook 7* (pp. 772–799). Beverly Hills, CA: Sage.

Larson, M. S. (1977). *The rise of professionalism: A sociological analysis*. Berkely, CA: University of California Press.

Lasswell, H. D. (1948). The structure and function of communication in society. In L. Bryson (Ed.), *The communication of ideas*. New York: Institute for Social and Religious Studies.

Lawrence, P. R., & Lorsch, J. W. (1967). *Organization and environment: Managing differentiation and integration*. Boston: Harvard Business School.

Lee, G. K., & Cole, R. E. (2003). From a firm-based to a community-based model of knowledge creation: The case of Linux kernel development. *Organization Science, 14*, 633–649.

Leiter, M. P. (1988). Burnout as a function of communication patterns: A study of a multidisciplinary mental health team. *Group and Organization Studies, 13*, 111–128.

Lenz, E. R. (1984). Information seeking: A component of client decisions and health behavior. *Advance in Nursing Science, 6*, 59–72.

Leonard, D. A. (2006). Innovation as a knowledge generation and transfer process. In A. Singhal & J. W. Dearing (Eds.), *Communication of innovations: A journey with Ev Rogers* (pp. 83–111). Thousand Oaks, CA: Sage.

Leonard-Barton, D., & Deschamps, I. (1988). Managerial influence in the implementation of new technology. *Management Science, 34*, 1252–1265.

Lerman, C., Hughes, C., Trock, B. J., Myers, R. E., Main, D., Bonney, A., . . . Lynch, H. T. (1999). Genetic testing in families with hereditary nonpolyposis colon cancer. *Journal of the American Medical Association, 281*, 1618–1622.

Lerman, C., Narod, S., Schulman, K., Hughes, C., Gomez-Caminero, A., Bonney, G., . . . Lynch, H. (1996). BRCA1 testing in families with hereditary breast-ovarian cancer: A prospective study of patient decision making and outcomes. *Journal of American Medical Association, 275*, 1885–1892.

Lerman, C., Seay, J., Balshem, A., & Audrain, J. (1995). Interest in genetic testing among first-degree relatives of breast cancer patients. *American Journal of Medical Genetics, 57*, 385–392.

Lesser, E., & Prusak, L. (2004). *Creating value with knowledge: Insights from the IBM Institute for Business Value*. New York: Oxford University Press.

Lesser, E. L., & Storck, J. (2004). Communities of practice and organizational performance. In E. Lesser & L. Prusak (Eds.), *Creating value with knowledge: Insights from the IBM institute for business value* (pp. 107–123). New York: Oxford University Press.

Leventhal, H., Safer, M. A., & Panagis, D. M. (1983). The impact of communications on the self-regulation of health belief, decisions and behavior. *Health Education Quarterly, 10*, 3–29.

Levine, J. M., & Moreland, R. L. (2004). Collaboration: The social context of theory development. *Personality and Social Psychology Review, 8*, 164–172.

Lichtenstein, E., & Glasgow, R. E. (1992). Smoking cessation: What have we learned over the past decade? *Journal of Counseling and Clinical Psychology, 60* (4), 518–527.

Lieberman, D. A. (2012). Digital games for health behavior change: Research, design, and future directions. In S. M. Noar & N. G. Harrington (Eds.), *eHealth applications: Promising strategies for behavior change* (pp. 164–193). New York: Routledge.

Lievrouw, L. A. (1994). Information resources and democracy: Understanding the paradox. *Journal of the American Society for Information Science, 45*, 350–357.

Lingard, L., Espin, S., Whyte, S., Regehr, G., Baker, G. R., Reznick, R., . . . Grober, E. (2004). Communication failures in the operating room: An observational classification of recurrent types and effects. *Quality and Safety in Health Care, 13*, 330–334. doi: 10.1136/qshc.2003.008425.

Littlejohn, S. W. (1989). *Theories of human communication* (3rd ed.). Belmont, CA: Wadsworth Publishing Company.

Littlejohn, S. W. (1992). *Theories of human communication* (4th ed.). Belmont, CA: Wadsworth Publishing.

Littlejohn, S. W., & Foss, K. A. (2011). *Theories of human communication* (10th ed.). Long Grove, IL: Waveland Press.

Lometti, G. E., Reeves, B., & Bybee, C. R. (1977). Investigating the assumptions of uses and gratifications research. *Communication Research, 4* (3), 321–338. doi: 10.1177/009365027700400305.

Lorenz, E. H. (1991). Neither friends nor strangers: Informal networks of subcontracting in French industry. In G. Thompson, J. Frances, R. Levacic & J. Mitchell (Eds.), *Markets, hierarchies and networks: The coordination of social life* (pp. 183–192). Newbury Park, CA: Sage.

Lowery, W., & Anderson, W. B. (2002). *The impact of Web use on the public perception of physicians.* Paper presented at the Association for Education in Journalism and Mass Communication, Miami Beach, FL.

Ludman, E. J., Curry, S. J., Hoffman, E., & Taplin, S. (1999, July/August). Women's knowledge and attitudes about genetic testing for breast cancer susceptibility. *Effective Clinical Practice, 2*, 158–162.

Lustria, M. L. A., Cortese, J., Noar, S. M., & Glueckauf, R. L. (2009). Computer-tailored health interventions delivered over the Web: Review and analysis of key components. *Patient Education and Counseling, 74*, 156–173. doi: 10.1016/j.pec.2008.08.023.

MacCrimmon, K. R., & Taylor, R. N. (1976). Decision making and problem solving. In M. D. Dunnette (Ed.), *Handbook of industrial and organizational psychology*. Chicago, IL: Rand McNally.

Macdonald, K. M. (1995). *The sociology of the professions.* Thousand Oaks, CA: Sage.

Malenka, D. J., Baron, J. A., Johansen, S., Wahrenberger, J. W., & Ross, J. (1993). The framing effect of relative and absolute risk. *Journal of General and Internal Medicine, 8*, 543–548.

Mangham, I. L. (1996). Some consequences of taking Gareth Morgan seriously. In D. Grant & C. Oswick (Eds.), *Metaphor and organizations* (pp. 21–36). Thousand Oaks, CA: Sage.

March, J. G. (1994). *A primer on decision making: How decisions happen.* New York: Free Press.

March, J. G., & Simon, H. A. (1958). *Organizations.* New York: John Wiley.

Marcus, A. C., Heimendinger, P., Wolfe, D., Fairclough, B. K., Rimer, B. K., Morra, M., . . . Wooldridge, J. (2001). A randomized trial of a brief intervention to increase fruit and vegetable intake: A replication study among callers to the CIS. *Preventive Medicine, 33*, 204–216.

Marshak, R. J. (1996). Metaphors, metaphoric fields and organizational change. In D. Grant & C. Oswick (Eds.), *Metaphor and organizations* (pp. 147–165). Thousand Oaks, CA: Sage.

Marteau, T. M., & Croyle, R. T. (1998). The new genetics: Psychological responses to genetic testing. *British Medical Journal, 316*, 693–697.

Marwell, G., & Schmitt, D. R. (1967). Dimensions of compliance gaining behavior: An empirical analysis. *Sociometry, 30*, 350–364.

Massey, V. (1986). Perceived susceptibility to breast cancer and practice of breast self-examination. *Nursing Research, 35*, 183–185.

Mauboussin, M. (2007). *More than you know: Finding financial wisdom in unconventional places.* New York: Columbia University Press.

May, S. K. (1993). A communication course in organizational paradigms and metaphors. *Communication Education, 42*, 234–254.

McCorkle, S., & Mills, J. L. (1992). Rowboat in a hurricane: Metaphors of interpersonal conflict management. *Communication Reports, 5* (2), 57–66.

McGrath, C., & Krackhardt, D. (2003). Network conditions for organizational change. *Journal of Applied Behavioral Science, 39*, 324–336.

McGuire, W. J. (1961). The effectiveness of supportive and refutational defenses in immunizing defenses. *Sociometry, 24*, 184–197.

McGuire, W. J. (1989). Theoretical foundations of campaigns. In R. E. Rice & C. K. Atkin (Eds.), *Public communication campaigns* (pp. 43–66). Newbury Park, CA: Sage.

McKinnon, S. M., & Bruns, W. J., Jr. (1992). *The information mosaic.* Boston: Harvard Business School Press.

McMillan, J. J., & Cheney, G. (1996). The student as consumer: The implications and limitations of a metaphor. *Communication Education, 45* (1), 1–15.

McPherson, M., Smith-Lovin, L., & Brashears, M. E. (2006). Social isolation in America: Changes in core discussion networks over two decades. *American Sociological Review, 71*, 353–375.

Meischke, H. W. J. (1991). *Using the Health Belief Model to predict breast cancer–related information seeking.* (Unpublished doctoral dissertation). Michigan State University, East Lansing.

Metoyer-Duran, C. (1993). Information gatekeepers. In M. E. Williams (Ed.), *Annual review of information science and technology* (Vol. 28, pp. 111–150). Medford, NJ: Learned Information.

Meyer, A. D. (1984). Mingling decision making metaphors. *Academy of Management Review, 9*, 6–17.

Mikhail, B. (1981). The Health Belief Model: A review and critical evaluation of the model, research, and practice. *Advances in Nursing Science, 4*, 65–82.

Milardo, R. M. (1983). Social networks and pair relationships: A review of substantive and measurement issues. *Sociology and Social Research, 68*, 1–18.

Mileti, D. S., & Beck, E. M. (1975). Communication in crises: Explaining evacuation symbolically. *Communication Research, 2*, 24–49. doi:10.1177/009365027500200102.

Miller, G. R. (1969). Human information processing: Some research guidelines. In R. J. Kibler & L. L. Barker (Eds.), *Conceptual frontiers in speech communication* (pp. 51–68). New York: Speech Communication Association.

Miller, K. I., Zook, E. G., & Ellis, B. H. (1989). Occupational difference in the influence of communication on stress and burnout in the workplace. *Management Communication Quarterly, 3* (2), 166–190.

Mohrman, S. A., Tenkasi, R. V., & Mohrman, A. M., Jr. (2003). The role of networks in fundamental organizational change: A grounded analysis. *Journal of Applied Behavioral Science, 39,* 301–323.

Mongalindan, J. P. (2012, October 8). Quant Junkies. *Fortune,* 49.

Monge, P. R., & Contractor, N. S. (2003). *Theories of communication networks.* New York: Oxford University Press.

More, E. (1990). Information systems: People issues. *Journal of Information Science, 16,* 311–320.

Morgan, G. (1986). *Images of organization.* Beverly Hills, CA: Sage.

Morgan, S. E., King, A. J., & Ivic, R. K. (2011). Using new technologies to enhance health communication research methodology. In T. L. Thompson & R. Parrott (Eds.), *The Routledge handbook of health communication* (2nd ed., pp. 578–592). New York: Routledge.

Morley, D. (1993). Active audience theory: Pendulums and pitfalls. *Journal of Communication, 43,* 13–19.

Mukherjee, S. (2010). *The emperor of all maladies: A biography of cancer.* New York: Scribner.

Mullen, P. D., Hersey, J. C., & Iverson, D. C. (1987). Health behavior models compared. *Social Science and Medicine, 24,* 973–981.

Myers, S. A., Shimotsu, S., & Claus, C. J. (2013). Understanding work group dynamics: Effectively getting people to work cohesively in small groups. In J. S. Wrench (Ed.), *Workplace communication for the 21st century: Tools and strategies that impact the bottom line* (pp. 243–270). Santa Barbara, CA: Praeger.

Napoli, P. M. (1999). The marketplace of ideas metaphor in communications regulation. *Journal of Communication, 49* (4), 151–169.

National Cancer Institute. (2003). *Changing the conversation: The nation's investment in cancer research.* Rockville, MD: National Cancer Institute.

National Institutes of Health. (2006, October 3). NIH launches national consortium to transform clinical research. Retrieved from http://www.nih.gov/news/pr/oct2006/ncrr-03.htm.

Nebus, J. (2006). Building collegial information networks: A theory of advice network generation. *Academy of Management Review, 31,* 615–637.

Nemcek, M. A. (1990). Health beliefs and preventive behavior: A review of the research literature. *AAOHN Journal, 38,* 127–138.

Noar, S. M. (2006). A 10-year retrospective of research in health mass media campaigns: Where do we go from here? *Journal of Health Communication, 11,* 21–42. doi: 10.1080/10810730500461059.

Noar, S. M., Banac, C. N., & Harris, M. S. (2007). Does tailoring matter? Meta-analytic review of tailored print health behavior change interventions. *Psychological Bulletin, 133* (4), 673–693. doi: 10.1037/0033-2909.133.4.673.

Noar, S. M., Palmgreen, P., & Zimmerman, R. S. (2009). Reflections on evaluating health communication campaigns. *Communication Methods and Measures, 3* (1), 105–114. doi: 10.1080/19312450902809730.

Noelle-Neumann, E. (1974). The spiral of silence. *Journal of Communication, 24,* 43–51.

O'Reilly, C. A., III. (1980). Individuals and information overload in organizations: Is more necessarily better? *Academy of Management Journal, 23,* 684–696.

O'Reilly, C. A., III, Chatham, J. A., & Anderson, J. C. (1987). Message flow and decision making. In F. M. Jablin, L. L. Putnam, K. H. Roberts & L. W. Porter (Eds.), *Handbook of organizational communication: An interdisciplinary perspective* (pp. 600–623). Newbury Park, CA: Sage.

O'Reilly, C. A., III, & Pondy, L. R. (1979). Organizational communication. In S. Kerr (Ed.), *Organizational behavior* (pp. 119–150). Columbus, OH: Grid.

Okhuysen, G. A., & Bechky, B. A. (2009). Coordination in organizations: An integrative perspective. *Academy of Management Annals, 3* (1), 463–502. doi: 10.1080/19416520903047533.

Oldenburg, B. F., Sallis, J. F., French, M. L., & Owen, N. (1999). Health promotion research and the diffusion and institutionalization of interventions. *Health Education Research, 14,* 121–130.

Orleans, C. T. (2005). The behavior change consortium: Expanding the boundaries and impact of health behavior change research. *Annals of Behavioral Medicine, 29,* 76–79.

Oswick, C., Fleming, P., & Hanlon, G. (2011). From borrowing to blending: Re-thinking the process of organizational theory building. *Academy of Management Review, 36* (2), 316–337.

Oswick, C., & Jones, P. (2006). Beyond correspondence? Metaphor in organization theory. *Academy of Management Review, 31,* 483–485.

Paddock, C. (2013). 7 in 10 Americans track health. *Medical News Today.* Retrieved from http://www.medicalnewstoday.com/articles/255531.php.

Paisley, W. (1994). New media and methods of health communication. In L. Sechrest, T. E. Backer, E. M. Rogers, T. F. Campbell & M. L. Grady (Eds.), *Effective dissemination of clinical and health information* (pp. 165–180). Rockville, MD: Agency for Health Care Policy Research, AHCPR Pub. No. 95-0015.

Palmer, I., & Dunford, R. (1996). Conflicting use of metaphors: Reconceptualizing their use in the field of organizational change. *Academy of Management Review, 21,* 691–717.

Palmgreen, P. (1984). Uses and gratifications: A theoretical perspective. In R. N. Bostrom (Ed.), *Communication yearbook 8* (pp. 20–55). Beverly Hills, CA: Sage.

Palmgreen, P., Donohew, L., Lorch, E. P., Hoyle, R. H., & Stephenson, M. T. (2002). Television campaigns and sensation seeking targeting adolescent marijuana use: A controlled time series approach. In R. C. Hornik (Ed.), *Public health communication: Evidence for behavior change* (pp. 35–56). Mahwah, NJ: Lawrence Earlbaum Associates.

Park, A. (2012, August 6). Web MDs: Social media are changing how we diagnose disease. *Time. www.time.com/time/magazine/0,9263,7601120806,00.html.*

Parks, M. R. (1982). Ideology in interpersonal communication: Off the couch and into the world. In M. Burgoon (Ed.), *Communication yearbook 5* (pp. 79–107). New Brunswick, NJ: Transaction Books.

Parks, M. R., & Adelman, M. B. (1983). Communication networks and the development of romantic relationships: An expansion of uncertainty reduction theory. *Human Communication Research, 10*, 55–79.

Parks, M. R., Stan, C. M., & Eggert, L. L. (1983). Romantic involvement and social network involvement. *Social Psychology Quarterly, 46*, 116–131.

Parrott, R., & Kreuter, M. W. (2011). Multidisciplinary, interdisciplinary, and transdisciplinary approaches to health communication. In T. L. Thompson, R. Parrott & J. F. Nussbaum (Eds.), *The Routledge handbook of health communication* (pp. 3–17). New York: Routledge.

Paulos, J. A. (1989). *Innumeracy: Mathematical illiteracy and its consequences.* New York: Hill and Wang.

Perry-Smith, J. E. (2006). Social yet creative: The role of social relationships in facilitating individual creativity. *Academy of Management Journal, 49*, 85–101.

Perry-Smith, J. E., & Shalley, C. E. (2003). The social side of creativity: A static and dynamic social network perspective. *Academy of Management Review, 28*, 89–106.

Perse, E. M., & Courtright, J. A. (1993). Normative images of communication media: Mass and interpersonal channels in the new media environment. *Human Communication Research, 19*, 485–503.

Petronio, S. (2002). *Boundaries of privacy: Dialectics of disclosure.* Albany: State University of New York Press.

Petronio, S., & Reierson, J. (2009). Regulating the privacy of confidentiality: Grasping the complexities through communication privacy management theory. In T. D. Afifi & W. A. Afifi (Eds.), *Uncertainty, information management, and disclosure decisions: Theories and applications* (pp. 365–383). New York: Routledge.

Petty, R. E., & Cacioppo, J. (1986). The elaboration likelihood model of persuasion. In L. Berkowitz (Ed.), *Advances in experimental social psychology* (pp. 123–205). San Diego: Academic Press.

Pfeffer, J., & Sutton, R. I. (2006). *Hard facts, dangerous half-truths and total nonsense: Profiting from evidence-based management.* Cambridge, MA: Harvard Business School Press.

Pfister, D. S., & Soliz, J. (2011). (Re)conceptualizing intercultural communication in a networked society. *Journal of International and Intercultural Communication, 4* (4), 246–252. doi: 10.1080/17513057.2011.598043.

Pirolli, P., & Card, S. (1999). Information foraging. *Psychological Review, 106*, 643–675.

Polanyi, M., & Prosch, H. (1975). *Meaning.* Chicago: University of Chicago Press.

Poole, M. S., & DeSanctis, G. (1992). Microlevel structuration in computer-supported group decision making. *Human Communication Research, 19* (1), 5–49.

Poole, M. S., & Real, K. (2003). Groups and teams in health care: Communication and effectiveness. In T. L. Thompson, A. M. Dorsey, K. I. Miller & R. Parrott (Eds.), *Handbook of Health Communication* (pp. 369–402). Mahwah, NJ: Lawrence Earlbaum Associates.

Powell, W. W. (1990). Neither market nor hierarchy: Network forms of organization. In S. B. Bacharach (Ed.), *Research in organizational behavior* (pp. 295–336). Norwich, CT: JAI Press.

Power, D. J. (2007). A brief history of decision support systems. Version 4.1. Decision Support Systems Resources. Retrieved March 10, 2007, from http://DSSResources.COM/history/dsshistory.html.

Prochaska, J. O., & DiClemente, C. C. (1983). Stage process of self-change of smoking: Toward an integrative model of change. *Journal of Consulting and Clinical Psychology, 51,* 390–395.

Prochaska, J. O., & DiClemente, C. C. (1985). Common processes of self-change of smoking, weight control, and psychological distress. In S. Shiffman & T. A. Wills (Eds.), *Coping and substance use* (pp. 345–363). New York: Academic Press.

Prochaska, J. O., & DiClemente, C. C. (1986). Toward a comprehensive model of change. In M. Hersen, R. M. Eisler & P. M. Miller (Eds.), *Progress in behavior modification* (pp. 3–27). New York: Plenum Press.

Prochaska, J. O., DiClemente, C. C., & Norcross, J. C. (1992). In search of how people change: Applications to addictive behaviors. *American Psychologist, 47,* 1102–1114.

Putnam, L. L. (2010). Communication as changing the negotiation game. *Journal of Applied Communication Research, 38* (4), 325–335. doi: 10.1080/00909882.2010.513999.

Putnam, L. L., & Boys, S. (2006). Revisiting metaphors of organizational communication. In S. R. Clegg, C. Hardy, T. B. Lawrence & W. Nord (Eds.), *Sage handbook of organization studies* (pp. 541–576). Thousand Oaks, CA: Sage.

Putnam, L. L., & Holmer, M. (1992). Framing, reframing, and issue development. In L. L. Putnam & M. E. Roloff (Eds.), *Communication and negotiation* (pp. 128–155). Newbury Park, CA: Sage.

Putnam, L. L., Phillips, N., & Chapman, P. (1996). Metaphors of communication and organization. In S. R. Clegg, C. Hardy & W. R. Nord (Eds.), *Handbook of organization studies* (pp. 375–408). Thousand Oaks, CA: Sage.

Putnam, R. D. (2000). *Bowling alone: The collapse and revival of American community.* New York: Simon & Schuster.

Quinlan, E. (2009). The "actualities" of knowledge work: An institutional ethnography of multi-disciplinary primary health care teams. *Sociology of Health and Illness, 31* (5), 625–641. doi: 10.1111/j.1467–9566.2009.01167.x.

Raghavan, S. (2005). Medical decision support systems and knowledge sharing standards. In R. K. Bali (Ed.), *Clinical knowledge management: Opportunities and challenges* (pp. 196–217). Hershey, PA: Idea Group Publishing.

Ramirez, A., Jr., & Wang, Z. (2008). When online meets offline: An expectancy violations theory perspective on modality switching. *Journal of Communication, 58,* 20–39.

Ray, E. B. (1987). Supportive relationships and occupational stress in the workplace. In T. L. Albrecht & M. B. Adelman (Eds.), *Communicating social support* (pp. 172–191). Newbury Park, CA: Sage.

Ray, E. B., & Apker, J. (2011). Stress, burnout, and supportive communication: A review of research in health organizations. In T. L. Thompson, R. Parrott & J. F. Nussbaum (Eds.), *The Routledge handbook of health communication* (2nd ed., pp. 428–440). New York: Routledge.

Reagans, R., & McEvily, B. (2003). Network structure and knowledge transfer: The effect of cohesion and range. *Administrative Science Quarterly, 48,* 240–267.

Real, K. (2008). Information seeking and workplace safety: A field application of the risk perception attitude framework. *Journal of Applied Communication Research, 36,* 339–359. doi: 10.1080/00909880802101763.

Real, K., & Street, R. L., Jr. (2009). Doctor-patient communication from an organizational perspective. In D. Brashers & D. Goldsmith (Eds.), *Communicating to manage health and illness* (pp. 65–90). New York: Routledge.

Reay, T., Berta, W., & Kahn, M. K. (2009). What's the evidence on evidence-based management? *Academy of Management Perspectives, 23* (4), 5–18.

Reddy, M. C., & Spence, P. R. (2008). Collaborative information seeking: A field study of a multidisciplinary patient care team. *Information Processing and Management, 44,* 242–255.

Reddy, M. J. (1979). The conduit metaphor—a case of frame conflict in our language about language. In A. Ortony (Ed.), *Metaphor and thought* (pp. 284–324). Cambridge: Cambridge University Press.

Rice, R. E., & Atkin, C. K. (1989). Preface: Trends in communication campaign research. In R. E. Rice & C. K. Atkin (Eds.), *Public communication campaigns* (pp. 7–11). Newbury Park, CA: Sage.

Richards, W. D. (1985). Data, models, and assumptions in network analysis. In R. D. McPhee & P. K. Tompkins (Eds.), *Organizational communication: Traditional themes and new directions* (pp. 109–128). Beverly Hills, CA: Sage.

Rico, R., Sanchez-Manzanares, M., Gil, F., & Gibson, C. (2008). Team implicit coordination processes: A team knowledge-based approach. *Academy of Management Review, 33,* 153–184.

Rifkin, E., & Bouwer, E. (2007). *The illusion of certainty: Health benefits and risk.* New York: Springer.

Riley, W. T., Rivera, D. E., Atienza, A. A., Nilsen, W., Allison, S. M., & Mermelstein, R. (2011). Health behavior models in the age of mobile interventions: Are our theories up to the task? *Translational Behavioral Medicine, 1* (1), 53–71.

Rimal, R. N. (2001). Perceived risk and self-efficacy as motivators: Understanding individuals' long-term use of health information. *Journal of Communication, 51* (4), 633–654.

Rimal, R. N., & Adkins, A. D. (2003). Using computers to narrowcast health messages: The role of audience segmentation, targeting, and tailoring in health promotion. In T. L. Thompson, A. M. Dorsey, K. I. Miller & R. Parrott (Eds.), *Handbook of health communication* (pp. 497–513). Mahwah, NJ: Lawrence Erlbaum Associates.

Rimal, R. N., Flora, J. A., & Schooler, C. (1999). Achieving improvements in overall health orientation: Effects of campaign exposure, information seeking, and health media use. *Communication Research, 26* (3), 322–348.

Rimer, B. K., Davis, S. W., Engstrom, P. F., Myers, R. E., & Rosan, J. R. (1988). Some reasons for compliance and noncompliance in a health maintenance organization breast cancer screening program. *Journal of Compliance with Health Care, 3,* 103–113.

Robertson, T. S., & Wortzel, L. H. (1977). Consumer behavior and health care change: The role of mass media. *Consumer Research, 4,* 525–527.

Rodgers, S., Chen, Q., Duffy, M., & Fleming, K. (2007). Media usage as health segmentation variables. *Journal of Health Communication, 12,* 105–119. doi: 10.1080/10810730601150064.

Rogers, E. M. (2003). *The diffusion of innovations* (5th ed.). New York: Free Press.

Rogers, E. M., & Adhikayra, R. (1979). Diffusion of innovations: An up-to-date review and commentary. In D. Nimmo (Ed.), *Communication yearbook 3* (pp. 67–81). New Brunswick, NJ: Transaction Books.

Rogers, E. M., & Storey, J. D. (1987). Communication campaigns. In C. R. Berger & S. H. Chaffee (Eds.), *Handbook of communication science* (pp. 817–846). Newbury Park, CA: Sage.

Rohrbach, L. A., Grana, R., Sussman, S., & Valente, T. W. (2006). Type II translation: Transporting prevention interventions from research to real-world settings. *Evaluation and the Health Professions, 29,* 302–333. doi: 10.1177/0163278706290408.

Rosenstock, I. M. (1974). The Health Belief Model and preventive health behavior. *Health Education Monographs, 2,* 354–386.

Rosenstock, I. M. (1990). The Health Belief Model: Explaining health behavior through expectancies. In K. Glanz, F. M. Lewis & B. K. Rimer (Eds.), *Health behavior and health education: Theory, research and practice* (pp. 36–92). San Francisco, CA: Jossey-Bass.

Rosenstock, I. M., Strecher, V. J., & Becker, M. (1988). Social learning theory and the Health Belief Model. *Health Education Quarterly, 15,* 175–183.

Roter, D. L., & Hall, J. A. (2011). How medical interaction shapes and reflects the physician-patient relationship. In T. L. Thompson, R. Parrott & J. F. Nussbaum (Eds.), *The Routledge handbook of health communication* (2nd ed., pp. 55–68). New York: Routledge.

Rothstein, M. A. (1997). Genetic secrets: A policy framework. In M. A. Rothstein (Ed.), *Genetic secrets: Protecting privacy and confidentiality in the genetic era* (pp. 451–495). New Haven, CT: Yale University Press.

Rousseau, D., & McCarthy, S. (2007). Educating managers from an evidence-based perspective. *Academy of Management Learning and Education, 6* (1), 84–101.

Rowley, J. E., & Turner, C. M. D. (1978). *The dissemination of information.* Boulder, CO: Westview Press.

Rubin, A. M. (1986). Uses, gratifications, and media effects research. In J. Bryant & D. Zillman (Eds.), *Perspectives on media effects* (pp. 281–301). Hillsdale, NJ: Lawrence Erlbaum Associates.

Rynes, S. L., Bartunek, J. M., & Daft, R. L. (2001). Across the great divide: Knowledge creation and transfer between practitioners and academics. *Academy of Management Journal, 44,* 340–355.

Sabee, C. M., Bylund, C. L., Weber, J. G., & Sonet, E. (2012). The association of patients' primary interaction goals with attributions for their doctors' responses in conversations about online health research. *Journal of Applied Communication Research, 40* (3), 271–288.

Salmon, C. T., & Atkin, C. (2003). Using media campaigns for health promotion. In T. L. Thompson, A. M. Dorsey, K. I. Miller & R. Parrott (Eds.), *Handbook of health communication* (pp. 449–472). Mahwah, NJ: Lawrence Erlbaum Associates.

Scarbrough, H., & Swan, J. (2002). Knowledge communities and innovation. *Trends in Communication, 8,* 7–18.

Schon, D. A. (1979). Generative metaphor: A perspective on problem-setting in social policy. In A. Ortony (Ed.), *Metaphor and thought* (pp. 254–283). Cambridge: Cambridge University Press.

Schon, D. A., & Rein, M. (1994). *Frame reflection: Toward the resolution of intractable policy controversies.* New York: Basic Books.

Schramm, W. (1972). The nature of communication between humans. In W. Schramm & D. F. Roberts (Eds.), *The process and effects of mass communication* (pp. 3–53). Urbana: University of Illinois Press.

Schwartz, B. (2004). *Paradox of choice: Why more is less.* New York: Harper Collins.

Schwartz, L. M., Woloshin, S., Black, W. C., & Welch, H. G. (1997). The role of numeracy in understanding the benefit of screening mammography. *Annals of Internal Medicine, 127* (11), 966–972.

Scott, J. (2000). *Social network analysis: A handbook* (2nd ed.). Thousand Oaks, CA: Sage.

Sears, D. O., & Freedman, J. L. (1967). Selective exposure to information: A critical review. *Public Opinion Quarterly, 31,* 194–213.

Seibold, D. R., & Roper, R. E. (1979). Psychosocial determinants of health care intentions: Test of the Triandis and Fishbein models. In D. Nimmo (Ed.), *Communication yearbook 3* (pp. 625–643). New Brunswick, NJ: Transaction Books.

Senge, P. M. (1990). *The fifth discipline: The art and practice of the learning organization.* New York: Doubleday Currency.

Shapiro, A. L. (1999). *The control revolution . . . : How the Internet is putting individuals in charge and changing the world we know.* New York: Public Affairs.

Shapiro, D. L., Kirkman, B. L., & Courtney, H. G. (2007). Perceived causes and solutions of the translation problem in management research. *Academy of Management Journal, 50* (2), 249–266.

Sharf, B., & Vanderford, M. L. (2003). Illness narratives and social construction of health. In T. L. Thompson, A. M. Dorsey, K. I. Miller & R. Parrott (Eds.), *Handbook of health communication.* Mawah, NJ: Lawrence Erlbaum.

Shaw, M. E. (1971). *Group dynamics: The psychology of small group behavior.* New York: McGraw-Hill.

Sheppard, S. L., Solomon, L. J., Atkins, E., Foster, R. S., Jr., & Frankowski, B. (1990). Determinants of breast self-examination among women of lower income and lower education. *Journal of Behavioral Medicine, 13,* 359–371.

Sherer, C. W., & Juanillo, N. K., Jr. (1992). Bridging theory and praxis: Reexamining public health communication. In S. A. Deetz (Ed.), *Communication yearbook 15* (pp. 312–345). Newbury Park, CA: Sage.

Sherif, M., & Sherif, C. W. (1964). *Reference groups: Exploration into conformity and deviation of adolescents.* Chicago: Henry Regnery.

Sicotte, C., D'Amour, D., & Moreault, M. (2002). Interdisciplinary collaboration within Quebec community health care centres. *Social Science and Medicine, 55,* 993–1003.

Sidransky, D. (1996, September). Advances in cancer detection. *Scientific American, 275,* 104–109.

Siefert, M., Gerbner, G., & Fisher, J. (1989). *The information gap: How computers and other new communication technologies affect the social distribution of power.* New York: Oxford University Press.

Silk, K. J., Atkin, C. K., & Salmon, C. T. (2011). Developing effective media campaigns for health promotion. In T. L. Thompson, R. Parrott & J. F. Nussbaum (Eds.), *The Routledge handbook of health communication* (pp. 203–219). New York: Routledge.

Silva, V. T. (2005). In the beginning was the gene: The hegemony of genetic thinking in contemporary culture. *Communication Theory, 15* (1), 100–123.

Simon, H. A. (1987). Making management decisions: The role of intuition and emotion. *Academy of Management Executive, 1,* 57–64.

Slater, M. D. (2004). Operationalizing and analyzing exposure: The foundation of media effects research. *Journalism and Mass Communication Quarterly, 81,* 168–183.

Slater, M. D., Hayes, A. F., Reineke, J. B., Long, M., & Bettinghaus, E. P. (2009). Newspaper coverage of cancer prevention: Multilevel evidence for knowledge gap affects. *Journal of Communication, 59,* 514–533.

Smircich, L., & Calas, M. B. (1987). Organizational culture: A critical assessment. In F. M. Jablin, L. L. Putnam, K. H. Roberts & L. W. Porter (Eds.), *Handbook of organizational communication: An interdisciplinary perspective* (pp. 228–263). Newbury Park, CA: Sage.

Smith, H. A., & McKeen, J. D. (2003). Creating and facilitating communities of practice. In C. W. Holsapple (Ed.), *Handbook of knowledge management 1: Knowledge matters* (pp. 393–407). New York: Springer-Verlag.

Smithson, M. (1989). *Ignorance and uncertainty: Emerging paradigms.* New York: Springer-Verlag.

Snyder, J. (2009). The role of coworker and supervisor social support in alleviating the experience of burnout for caregivers in the human-services industry. *Southern Communication Journal, 74* (4), 373–389. doi: 10.1080/10417940802516834.

Snyder, L. B., & Hamilton, M. A. (2002). A meta-analysis of US health campaign effects on behavior: Emphasize enforcement, exposure, and new information and beware the secular trend. In R. C. Hornik (Ed.), *Public health communication: Evidence for behavior change.* Mahwah, NJ: Lawrence Erlbaum Associates.

Sontag, S. (1978). *Illness as metaphor.* New York: Farrar, Straus, and Giroux.

Sontag, S. (1988). *AIDS and its metaphors.* New York: Farrar, Straus, and Giroux.

Sopory, P., & Dillard, J. P. (2002). The persuasive effects of metaphor: A meta-analysis. *Human Communication Research, 28* (3), 382–419.

Stafford, L. (2003). Maintaining romantic relationships: A summary and analysis of one research program. In D. J. Canary & M. Dainton (Eds.), *Maintaining relationships through communication: Relational, contextual, and cultural variations* (pp. 51–78). Mahwah, NJ: Lawrence Erlbaum Associates.

Stafford, L. (2005). *Maintaining long-distance and cross-residential relationships.* Mahwah, NJ: Lawrence Erlbaum.

Stafford, L., & Canary, D. J. (1991). Maintenance strategies and romantic relationship type, gender and relational characteristics. *Journal of Social and Personal Relationships, 8,* 217–242. doi: 10.1177/0265407591082004.

Stasser, G., & Titus, W. (1985). Pooling of unshared information in group decision making: Biased information sampling during discussion. *Journal of Personality and Social Psychology, 48*, 1467–1478.

Staw, B. M., Sandelands, L. E., & Dutton, J. E. (1981). Threat rigidity effects in organizational behavior: A multilevel analysis. *Administrative Science Quarterly, 26*, 501–524.

Stephenson, M. T., Southwell, B. G., & Yzer, M. (2011). Advancing health comunication research: Issues and controversies in research design and data analysis. In T. L. Thompson, R. Parrott & J. F. Nussbaum (Eds.), *The Routledge handbook of health communication* (2nd ed., pp. 560–577). New York: Routledge.

Stewart, T. A. (2001). *The wealth of knowledge: Intellectual capital and the twenty-first century organization.* New York: Currency.

Stohl, C., & Redding, W. C. (1987). Messages and message exchange processes. In F. M. Jablin, L. L. Putnam, K. H. Roberts & L. W. Porter (Eds.), *Handbook of organizational communication: An interdisciplinary perspective* (pp. 451–502). Newbury Park, CA: Sage.

Stokols, D. (2006). Toward a science of transdisciplinary action research. *American Journal of Community Psychology, 38*, 63–77. doi: 10.1007/s10464-006-9060-5.

Stopfer, J. E. (2000). Genetic counseling and clinical cancer genetics services. *Seminars in Surgical Oncology 2000, 18*, 347–357.

Su, C., Huang, M., & Contractor, N. (2010). Understanding the structures, antecedents and outcomes of organisational learning and knowledge transfer: A multitheoretical and multilevel network analysis. *European Journal of International Management, 4* (6), 576–601.

Sundar, S. S., Rice, R. E., Kim, H., & Sciamanna, C. N. (2011). Online health information: Conceptual challenges and theoretical opportunities. In T. L. Thompson, R. Parrott & J. F. Nussbaum (Eds.), *The Routledge handbook of health communication* (2nd ed., pp. 181–202). New York: Routledge.

Sweeney, K. (2006). Personal knowledge: Doctors are much more than simple conduits for clinical evidence. *British Medical Journal, 332*, 129–130.

Szulanski, G. (1996). Exploring internal stickiness: Impediments to the transfer of best practice within the firm. *Strategic Management Journal, 17*, 27–43.

Szulanski, G. (2003). *Sticky knowledge: Barriers to knowing in the firm.* Thousand Oaks, CA: Sage.

Tan, A. S. (1985). *Mass communication theories and research.* New York: Wiley.

Taylor, H., & Leitman, R. (2002). Four-nation survey shows widespread but different levels of Internet use for health purposes. *Health Care News*, from http://www.harrisinteractive.com/newsletters_healthcare.asp.

Taylor, M. (1968). Towards a mathematical theory of influence and attitude change. *Human Relations, 98*, 128–139.

Tenkasi, R. V., & Chesmore, M. C. (2003). Social networks and planned organizational change: The impact of strong network ties on effective change implementation and use. *Journal of Applied Behavioral Science, 39*, 281–300.

Thayer, L. (1988). How does information "inform." In B. D. Ruben (Ed.), *Information and behavior* (Vol. 2, pp. 13–26). New Brunswick, NJ: Transaction Books.

Thompson, J. D. (1967). *Organizations in action*. New York: McGraw-Hill.

Thompson, T. G., & Brailer, D. J. (2004). *The decade of health information technology: Delivering consumer-centric and information-rich health care*. Rockville, MD: Health and Human Services.

Thompson, T. L. (2003). Introduction. In T. L. Thompson, A. M. Dorsey, K. I. Miller & R. Parrott (Eds.), *Handbook of Health Communication* (pp. 1–5). Mahwah, NJ: Lawrence Erlbaum Associates.

Tichenor, P. J., Donohue, G. A., & Olien, C. N. (1970). Mass media and differential growth in knowledge. *Public Opinion Quarterly, 34*, 158–170.

Tidd, J. (2000). The competence cycle: Translating knowledge into new processes, products, and services. In J. Tidd (Ed.), *From knowledge management to strategic competence: Measuring technological, market, and organizational innovation* (pp. 5–25). London: Imperial College Press.

Turner, M. M., Skubisz, C., & Rimal, R. N. (2011). Theory and practice in risk communication: A review of the literature and visions of the future. In T. L. Thompson, R. Parrott & J. F. Nussbaum (Eds.), *The Routledge handbook of health communication* (2nd ed., pp. 146–164). New York: Routledge.

Tustin, N. (2010). The role of patient satisfaction in online health information seeking. *Journal of Health Communication, 15*, 3–17. doi: 10.1080/108107309003465491.

Tversky, A., & Kahneman, D. (1981). The framing of decisions and the psychology of choice. *Science, 211*, 453–458.

Uzzi, B., & Spiro, J. (2005). Collaboration and creativity: The small world problem. *American Journal of Sociology, 111*, 447–504.

Valente, T. (2006). Communication network analysis and the diffusion of innovations. In A. Singhal & J. W. Dearing (Eds.), *A journey with Ev Rogers* (pp. 61–82). Thousand Oaks, CA: Sage.

Valente, T. W. (1995). *Network models of the diffusion of innovations*. Cresskill, NJ: Hampton Press.

Van de Ven, A. (2000). The president's message: The practice of management knowledge. *Academy of Management News, 31*, 4–5.

Van de Ven, A. (2002). Strategic directions for the Academy of Management: This academy is for you! *Academy of Management Review, 27*, 171–184.

Van de Ven, A. H. (1986). Central problems in the management of innovation. *Management Science, 32*, 590–607.

Van den Bulte, C., & Lillien, G. L. (2001). Medical innovation revisited: Social contagion versus marketing effort. *American Journal of Sociology, 106*, 1409–1435.

Van der Krogt, F. J. (1998). Learning network theory: The tension between learning systems and work systems in organizations. *Human Resource Development Quarterly, 9*, 157–177.

Varan, D. (1998). The cultural erosion metaphor and the transcultural impact of media systems. *Journal of Communication, 48* (2), 58–85.

Vaughan, D. (1999). The dark side of organizations: Mistake, misconduct, and disaster. *Annual Review of Sociology, 25*, 271–305.

Victor, B., & Blackburn, R. S. (1987). Interdependence: An alternative conceptualization. *Academy of Management Review, 12*, 486–498.

Viswanath, K., Kahn, E., Finnegan, J. R., Jr., Hertog, J., & Potter, J. D. (1993). Motivation and the knowledge gap: Effects of a campaign to reduce diet-related cancer risk. *Communication Research, 20*, 546–563.

von Hayek, F. (1991). Spontaneous ("grown") order and organized ("made") order. In G. Thompson, J. Frances, R. Levacic & J. Mitchell (Eds.), *Markets, hierarchies, and networks: The coordination of social life* (pp. 293–301). Newbury Park, CA: Sage.

von Hayek, F. A. (1945). The uses of knowledge in society. *American Economic Review, 35*, 519–520.

Wahlin, T. R. (2007). To know or not to know: A review of behaviour and suicidal ideation in preclinical Huntington's disease. *Patient Eduation and Counseling, 65*, 279–287.

Wakefield, M. A., Loken, B., & Hornik, R. C. (2010). Use of mass media campaigns to change health behaviors. *Lancet, 376*, 1261–1271.

Walker, K. L., & Stohl, C. (2012). Communicating in a collaborating group: A longitudinal network analysis. *Communication Monographs, 79* (4), 448–474. doi: 10.1080/03637751.2012.723810.

Wandersman, A., Goodman, R. M., & Butterfoss, F. D. (1997). Understanding coalitions and how they operate: An "open systems" organizational framework. In M. Minkler (Ed.), *Community organizing and community building for health* (pp. 261–277). New Brunswick, NJ: Rutgers University Press.

Ward, S. (1987). Consumer behavior. In C. R. Berger & S. H. Chaffee (Eds.), *Handbook of communication science* (pp. 651–674). Newbury Park, CA: Sage.

Wardle, F. J., Collins, W., Pernet, A. L., Whitehead, M. I., Bourne, T. H., & Campbell, S. (1993). Psychological impacts of screening for familial ovarian cancer. *Journal of the National Cancer Institute, 85* (8), 653–657.

Watts, D. J. (2002). A simple model of global cascades on random networks. *PNAS, 99*, 5766–5771.

Watts, D. J. (2003). *Six degrees: The science of the connected age*. New York: W. W. Norton.

Welkenhuysen, M., Evers-Kiebooms, G., Decruyensaere, M., Claes, E., & Denayer, L. (2001). A community based study on intentions regarding predictive testing for hereditary breast cancer. *Journal of Medical Genetics, 38*, 540–547.

Wenger, E., McDermott, R., & Snyder, W. M. (2002). *Cultivating communities of practice: A guide to managing knowledge*. Boston: Harvard Business School Press.

West, E., Barron, D. N., Dowsett, J., & Newton, J. N. (1999). Hierarchies and cliques in social networks of health care professionals: Implications for the design of dissemination strategies. *Social Science and Medicine, 48*, 633–646.

Wicks, P., Massagli, M., Frost, J., Brownstein, C., Okun, S., Vaughan, T., . . . Heywood, J. (2010). Sharing health data for better outcomes on PatientsLikeMe. *Journal of Medical Internet Research, 12* (2). Retrieved from http://www.jmir.org/2010/2/e19. doi:10.2196/jmir.1549.

Wilensky, H. L. (1968). Organizational intelligence. In D. L. Sills (Ed.), *The international encyclopedia of the social sciences* (pp. 319–334). New York: Free Press.

Witte, K. (1992). Putting the fear back into fear appeals: The extended parallel process model. *Communication Monographs, 59*, 329–349.

Witte, K. (1994). Fear control and danger control: A test of the Extended Parallel Process Model (EPPM). *Communication Monographs, 61*, 113–134.

Woelful, J., Cody, M. J., Gillham, J., & Holmes, R. A. (1980). Basic premises of multidimensional attitude change theory: An experimental analysis. *Academy of Management Journal, 6*, 153–167.

Wolgemuth, L. (2009, July). Beyond nursing: Hot healthcare jobs. *US News & World Report, 45*.

Wood, J. T., & Phillips, G. M. (1980). Metaphysical metaphors and pedagogical practices: Biological beings, pawns, interchangeable components, puppets, and hunting packs. *Communication Education, 29*, 146–157.

Wood, M. L. M. (2007). Rethinking the inoculation analogy: Effects on subjects with differing pre-existing attitudes. *Human Communication Research, 33*, 357–378.

Woodward, J. (1965). *Industrial organization*. London: Oxford University Press.

World Health Organization. (2003). *Adherence to long-term therapies: Evidence for action*. Geneva: World Health Organization.

Wright, K. B., Frey, L., & Sopory, P. (2007). Willingness to communicate about health as an underlying trait of patient self-advocacy: The development of the willingness to communicate about health (WTCH) measure. *Communication Studies, 58* (1), 35–51.

Wright, K. B., Johnson, A. J., Bernard, D. R., & Averbeck, J. (2011). Computer-mediated social support: Promises and pitfalls for individuals coping with health concerns. In T. L. Thompson, R. Parrott & J. F. Nussbaum (Eds.), *The Routledge handbook of health communication* (pp. 349–362). New York: Routledge.

Wright, K. B., Sparks, L., & O'Hair, H. D. (2008). *Health communication in the 21st century*. Malden, MA: Blackwell.

Zaltman, G. (1994). Knowledge disavowal in organizations. In R. H. Kilmann, K. W. Thomas, D. P. Slevin, R. Nath & S. L. Jerrell (Eds.), *Producing useful knowledge in organizations* (pp. 173–187). San Francisco: Jossey-Bass.

Zarit, S., & Femia, E. (2008). Behavioral and psychosocial interventions for family caregivers. *American Journal of Nursing, 108* (9), 47–53.

Zimbardo, P. G. (1960). Involvement and communication discrepancy as determinants of opinion conformity. *Journal of Abnormal and Social Psychology, 60*, 86–94.

Zimmerman, S., Sypher, B. D., & Haas, J. W. (1996). A communication metamyth in the workplace: The assumption that more is better. *Journal of Business Communication, 33*, 185–204.

Index

About the Author

J. David Johnson is professor in the Department of Communication at the University of Kentucky. He is the author of seven other books: *Cancer-related Information Seeking*, *Information Seeking*, *Organizational Communication Structure*, *Innovation and Knowledge Management*, *Managing Knowledge Networks*, *Managerial Communication*, and *Health Information Seeking* with Donald Case.